Praise for Leslie Beck

"Canada's nutrition guru has mapped out a plan that guarantees a new you. If you follow her 12-week plan, you will lose weight. Period."
—*Calgary Herald*

"One of the more sensible 'diet' books out there."
—*The Georgia Straight*

"Beck's advice is straightforward, simple and realistic, and is supported by her years of experience in the weight-loss field."
—*Canadian Living*

"Read this book and change your life. *The No-Fail Diet* is more than a 'diet book.' It is a healthy, balanced way of eating. And it is a plan that will work for today and for years ahead."
—*Perspectives* health and wellness newsletter, McMaster University

"Leslie Beck offers indispensable advice for healthy living."
—James F. Balch, M.D.

"If you'd like to eat more healthfully, Leslie Beck is a must-read."
—*Homemakers*

"An easy-to-read, practical tool to help you on the path to healthier living."
—*Toronto Star*

"This book should be in every home in North America."
—Christiane Northrup, M.D.

"This book is invaluable."
—Chris Carmichael, personal coach to seven-time Tour de France champion Lance Armstrong, and author of *Chris Carmichael's Food for Fitness*

PENGUIN CANADA

THE NO-FAIL DIET

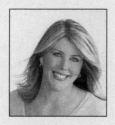

LESLIE BECK, a registered dietitian, is a leading Canadian nutritionist and the bestselling author of eight nutrition books. Leslie writes a weekly nutrition column in *The Globe and Mail*, is a regular contributor to CTV's *Canada AM*, and can be heard one morning a week on CJAD's *The Andrew Carter Show*.

Leslie has worked with many of Canada's leading businesses and international food companies, and runs a thriving private practice at the Medcan Clinic in Toronto. She also regularly delivers nutrition workshops to corporate groups across North America.

Visit Leslie Beck's website at **www.lesliebeck.com**.

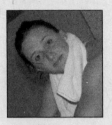

TRINA D. LAMBE, ACE, PT, RMT, is a certified personal trainer, spinning instructor, and massage therapist who owns an Ontario-wide agency of personal trainers who come to your home. She has been an active person all her life, initially as a national-level figure skater and now as a mountain biker. As a fitness expert, Trina can be heard on radio and is a regular guest on television health shows.

Also by Leslie Beck

Leslie Beck's Nutrition Encyclopedia

Leslie Beck's Nutrition Guide for Women

Leslie Beck's Nutrition Guide to a Healthy Pregnancy

Healthy Eating for Preteens and Teens

10 Steps to Healthy Eating

The Complete Nutrition Guide to Menopause

Foods That Fight Disease

The Easy
4-Step
Plan for
Permanent
Weight Loss

Leslie Beck RD

The No-Fail Diet

Recipe development and nutritional analysis:
Michelle Gelok, BASc

PENGUIN
CANADA

PENGUIN CANADA

Published by the Penguin Group

Penguin Group (Canada), 90 Eglinton Avenue East, Suite 700, Toronto, Ontario, Canada
M4P 2Y3 (a division of Pearson Canada Inc.)

Penguin Group (USA) Inc., 375 Hudson Street, New York, New York 10014, U.S.A.
Penguin Books Ltd, 80 Strand, London WC2R 0RL, England
Penguin Ireland, 25 St Stephen's Green, Dublin 2, Ireland (a division of Penguin Books Ltd)
Penguin Group (Australia), 250 Camberwell Road, Camberwell, Victoria 3124, Australia
(a division of Pearson Australia Group Pty Ltd)
Penguin Books India Pvt Ltd, 11 Community Centre, Panchsheel Park, New Delhi – 110 017,
India
Penguin Group (NZ), 67 Apollo Drive, Rosedale, North Shore 0632, New Zealand
(a division of Pearson New Zealand Ltd)
Penguin Books (South Africa) (Pty) Ltd, 24 Sturdee Avenue, Rosebank, Johannesburg 2196,
South Africa

Penguin Books Ltd, Registered Offices: 80 Strand, London WC2R 0RL, England

First published in 2006 by Penguin Group (Canada), a division of Pearson Canada Inc.
Published in this edition, 2008

3 4 5 6 7 8 9 10 (WEB)

Copyright © Leslie Beck, 2006
Exercise photos copyright © Trina Lambe, 2006
Photos of plates on page 16 courtesy of iDesign® Inc.

This publication contains the opinions and ideas of its author and is designed to provide useful
advice in regard to the subject matter covered. The author and publisher are not engaged
in rendering health or other professional services in this publication. This publication is not
intended to provide a basis for action in particular circumstances without consideration by
a competent professional. The author and publisher expressly disclaim any responsibility
for any liability, loss or risk, personal or otherwise, that is incurred as a consequence,
directly or indirectly, of the use and application of any of the contents of this book.

Manufactured in Canada.

Library and Archives Canada Cataloguing in Publication data available upon request

ISBN-10: 0-14-316763-4
ISBN-13: 978-0-14-316763-1

Visit the Penguin Group (Canada) website at **www.penguin.ca**

Special and corporate bulk purchase rates available; please see
www.penguin.ca/corporatesales or call 1-800-810-3104, ext. 2477 or 2474

Contents

Acknowledgments

I would like to thank the many people whose hard work, encouragement, and support made this book possible.

My researcher, Michelle Gelok, who contributed an enormous amount of time and energy to this book in writing the menu plans, developing and testing recipes, and compiling all of the nutrient analyses. I am incredibly grateful for her thoroughness and commitment to this project. I am also thankful to Michelle's mother, Gia Gelok, who loaned us the use of her kitchen for recipe testing.

My personal trainer, Trina Lambe, who developed the No-Fail 12-Week Fitness Program and who was always happy to answer my fitness-related questions. Her enthusiasm, energy, and incredible level of physical fitness are inspirations to me.

My private practice clients, who provided the inspiration for writing this book. Working with my clients over the years has allowed me to grow professionally and develop the tools and skills I use every day to help people achieve their nutrition goals.

My editors and the production team at Penguin Group (Canada) who encouraged me to put into words the approach and tools I use with clients to help them successfully lose weight.

My team, Dawn Bone, Rosemary Chubb, and Michelle Gelok, whose dedication, professionalism, and valuable inputs enable me to operate a successful private practice. I could not have accomplished all that I have without their assistance, hard work, and friendship. They truly are the foundation that supports my practice.

My family and friends, especially Darrell, who never waiver in their support of my work. Thank you for always cheering me on—and helping me stay balanced.

Introduction

According to Health Canada, at least 40% of women and almost 25% of all men are trying to lose weight. Efforts to lose weight start young too—among 12 to 14 year olds, 27% of girls and 14% of boys say they are trying to lose a few pounds. If you read the news reports, you'll know there's good reason for many Canadians to embark on a weight-loss program. According to the most recent statistics, 59% of the population is overweight or obese, a number that has steadily increased for almost every age group over the past 25 years.

If you're like many of my clients, chances are you have tried at least one weight-loss diet in the past. And in all likelihood, you've attempted one or two diets that failed. Perhaps they didn't help you lose very much weight because they were too hard to stick to. Or maybe you achieved your weight-loss goal, only to gain back the pounds you lost once you stopped the diet. The fact is that many diets do fail when it comes to helping people permanently lose weight. Any diet that's hard to follow, doesn't fit into real life, drastically cuts calories or entire food groups, makes you feel hungry and deprived, or doesn't change your core habits won't work over the long term. And too often diets are associated with feelings of guilt. People view harmless lapses as signs of failure and abandon their diet.

Keep in mind that diet is only part of the weight-loss equation, albeit a large part. Lifetime weight management is not just about what you eat. It requires physical activity as well. Regular exercise helps your body burn more calories (and allows you to enjoy more foods while you lose weight), and it is absolutely crucial for maintaining your weight loss.

I have spent my career as a registered dietitian helping people change their eating habits to successfully lose weight. I've done this by listening to my clients and understanding what's wrong with their diets and what needs fixing. I've designed hundreds of meal plans for my clients that help them lose weight, have more energy, consume more vitamins and minerals, and not feel hungry. Clients who consult me for weight loss eat at least four times per day and don't have to give up their favourite foods. They are able to eat real foods—the same foods that the rest of their family eats. In a nutshell, I give my clients what they ask me for—a practical, real-life plan that's easy to follow whether they're eating at home, in a restaurant, or in someone else's home. And that's why it works. My clients don't feel deprived on the diets I design for them. In fact, they tell me they feel more energetic and healthier than ever.

What Is the No-Fail Diet?

After writing six books—on subjects ranging from menopause to pregnancy to nutrition for teenagers—I decided it was time to put pen to paper and make the tools and tricks I offer my clients available to a wider audience. The No-Fail Diet is the result. It's my weight-loss plan that incorporates education about healthy eating, portion control strategies, and exercise advice. It's a plan that emphasizes four key factors to successful (that means permanent) weight loss: eating at the right times, including protein at meals, learning appropriate portion sizes, and tracking your progress. These four keys, plus regular physical activity, have helped my clients successfully manage their weight.

I've called it the No-Fail Diet because it's a way of eating that sets you up for success. Eating every 3 to 4 hours prevents you from becoming too hungry and overeating. Ensuring that your meals include a healthy protein food helps to slow down digestion and prolongs the satiety power of the diet. Learning what constitutes proper portion sizes of various foods helps you visualize what your meals should look like on your plate, making it easy to eat healthfully when you're away from home. Tracking your progress by keeping a food diary and documenting your body measurements helps motivate you to keep going. And finally, adding regular physical activity to your life boosts your motivation to make healthy food choices and helps keep the weight off once you've reached your goal.

But don't get me wrong. Just because I have called my plan the No-Fail Diet doesn't mean you won't slip from time to time. It is only natural to fall off track occasionally, but that does *not* mean you have failed. Lapses are a normal part of losing weight. The key is learning to get back on track quickly. By telling yourself it's okay to lapse, you give yourself permission to make a few mistakes along the way. It's that attitude that makes it easy to resume the No-Fail Diet—and succeed!

Phase 1, the Quick Start

Some people like to see results quickly when they are starting a weight-loss program. It helps them keep motivated. That's why I have included an *optional* 2-week Quick Start meal plan. This phase provides a meal plan that is a little stricter than that for the remaining weeks on the No-Fail Diet. It's entirely up to you whether you decide to follow the 2-week Quick Start meal plan. If you decide to skip it, you'll start instead at Phase 2.

Phase 2, Sustaining Weight Loss

The foundation of the No-Fail Diet includes four meal plans, each specifying a certain calorie level. You'll find a 1200-, 1400-, 1700-, and 2000-calorie meal plan. Which meal plan you choose will depend on your gender (men need more calories than women), your current weight (heavier bodies require more calories), and your activity level. You'll learn how to choose the one that's right for you.

Each meal plan is designed to help you eat a nutritionally balanced diet that includes foods from all food groups (yes, carbohydrates are allowed). The plans are designed to help you reduce your intake of saturated and trans fats and increase your intake of fibre, vitamins, minerals, and antioxidants. For each meal plan, I have spread your daily food servings over the course of the day to keep you feeling satisfied and energetic.

To help you follow the No-Fail Diet, you'll also find a 6-week menu plan that includes over 75 recipes, all of which have been nutritionally analyzed. If you don't want to follow a structured menu plan, feel free to pick and choose the meal and snack ideas that appeal to you and add them to your own repertoire of healthy meals. Once you know the structure of the No-Fail Diet meal plan, and the serving sizes of the foods you'll eat, it's easy to follow the plan with your own meal ideas.

Phase 3, Maintaining Your Weight Loss

When you reach your weight goal, you might need to adjust your food intake to prevent further weight loss. In Phase 3 of the No-Fail Diet, you'll learn what types of food to add back—and in what quantities—to stabilize your weight. You'll also learn 10 important strategies that will help you maintain your weight over the years to come.

The No-Fail 12-Week Fitness Program

I have devoted an entire chapter to physical activity and its importance in helping you achieve a healthy weight and overall well-being. You'll learn what type of exercise is best for losing body fat, how much you should do, and how hard you should work out. It might be as simple as adding four power walks to your weekly routine. Or you might need to boost the intensity on the cardio machine at the gym. In essence, I encourage you to do whatever works for you.

If you're really keen to improve your overall fitness level, you'll find a detailed No-Fail 12-Week Fitness Program designed by my personal trainer, Trina Lambe. Trina's 12-week program is designed to strengthen your entire body—your heart and lungs, the muscles in your upper and lower body, and the muscles that stabilize your spine (your core muscles). Each week it includes four cardio workouts, three strength-training workouts, and stretching exercises. Every 3 weeks, you will be given a new series of exercises to help you build your endurance and strength.

Your Personal Tracking Tools

Monitoring your progress is an important part of successful weight loss. That's why I have included tracking tools for you to use while you follow the No-Fail Diet. In Appendix 1 you'll find a Daily Food and Activity Tracker, a 12-Week Body Measurement Tracker, and a 12-Week Fitness Tracker (to use should you embark on the fitness program outlined in Chapter 5). I encourage you to make photo-copies of these tools so you'll have plenty of copies to see you through your program. If you prefer to track your progress online, you'll find the Daily Food and Activity Tracker and the Body Measurement Tracker on my website—www.lesliebeck.com. Just click on the No-Fail Diet.

IT'S NOW TIME to get started. It's time to assess your weight-loss readiness, set your own personal goals, and start thinking for success. The chapters that follow will give you the tools and information you need to achieve and maintain a weight that's healthy for you. It doesn't matter if it takes you one month, six months, or one year to reach your ultimate weight-loss goal. This is not a race. This is not a diet with a start point and end point. Rather, it's a way of eating that you can follow for the rest of your life. It's a plan that will help you make *permanent* changes to your eating and exercise habits that will promote weight loss and health—changes that you can sustain over the long term. Enjoy the journey.

Leslie Beck, RD

1

Getting Ready to Start the No-Fail Diet

It's hard to ignore the news stories that constantly tell us we're becoming a nation of overweight and obese people. Certainly, the statistics are worrisome. Today, 64% of North Americans are considered to be overweight or obese—that's two-thirds of the population.

Why have we become such a flabby nation? Figuring out the answer isn't rocket science: We eat too much and we move too little. We have easy access to huge portions of overly processed foods. Portion sizes are ridiculous in North America. Since the 1960s, portion sizes of foods sold in stores and restaurants—from chocolate bars to burgers and soft drinks—have become much bigger. Fast-food restaurants offer "king size" meal combos, muffins and bagels have doubled and tripled in size, and family-style restaurants serve pasta meals that could serve a family of four.

We're a sedentary bunch, too. Most of us don't accumulate the recommended 1 hour of daily physical activity. Don't get me wrong. I'm not saying we're lazy. Sure, some of us might lack the motivation to exercise or complain that there just isn't enough time, but there are other stumbling blocks that prevent us from being active. Our modern lifestyle predisposes us to becoming fat. We have jobs that require us to sit all day long. We rely on cars to take us—and our kids—everywhere. Many of us live in suburbs so sprawling that biking or walking to work, school, or the grocery store simply isn't an option.

Despite these environmental influences on our weight, being overweight is *not* inevitable. If you are overweight now, it is absolutely possible to lose those excess pounds. If you're like many of my clients, chances are you've made past attempts at weight loss. Perhaps you've even followed a fad diet and lost weight. But how long did you keep those pounds from creeping back on? Four weeks? Six months? One year?

Over the years, I have worked with many clients who told me they managed to lose weight by following one diet or another. Many said they were able to stick to the particular diet for its duration. Others told me that their diet was just too much work and so gave up partway through. Regardless of how many pounds were lost, people inevitably regained most of their weight loss, and sometimes more. Usually all it takes is for life to get in the way and throw people off course—a string of family birthday parties, a week of business travel, stress on the job, or conflict at home. Most people are pretty good at losing weight. Where we fall down is in maintaining a weight loss. If you've experienced that familiar post-diet weight gain, it's not because you failed the diet. It's because most diets fail people.

The problem with fad diets—diets that sell the fantasy that this time it will be different—is that they are often unbalanced. They make you feel hungry, they set up unrealistic expectations about what you can achieve, and they don't fit into real life. They don't teach you how to deal with family celebrations, vacations, and dining out. Fad diets make you feel guilty: You're either "on" or "off" the diet. When you're on, you tell yourself you're being good, and when you slip up, you berate yourself for being bad. And most fad diets don't tell you how to maintain your new figure once the weight-loss phase is over. The bottom line: Fad diets cannot be sustained.

The low-carb craze is a recent example of a fad diet that fell out of favour because it didn't offer a long-term solution to weight control. The low-carb diet exploded in the 1990s and remained popular until 2004, when dieters became concerned for their health and incredibly bored of bacon and eggs, bunless burgers, and countless cheese sticks. Sure enough, in 2005 we witnessed the demise of an era in which millions of North Americans adopted high-protein diets packed with meat and cheese, and shunned breads, pasta, rice, fruit, and milk in an effort to shed weight.

But even so-called good diets can fail if you're not ready to make them work. To succeed, you need to be ready to make some permanent changes to your eating and exercise habits. (Later in this chapter you'll find a quiz to help you determine your state of weight-loss readiness.) Once you've decided that the time is right to make a change, you need the proper tools to help you permanently lose weight. That's where the No-Fail Diet comes in.

The No-Fail Diet is designed to help you lose weight and keep it off. But let me be clear on one point: I am not promising miraculous results overnight. Sure, we would all love that magic bullet to help us shed weight quickly and effortlessly. But the truth is, being successful at weight loss—that means keeping the pounds off for good—requires motivation, the right attitude, and yes, hard work. The No-Fail Diet gives you the tools you need to help you succeed at getting to a weight that's right for your body and your lifestyle.

Are You Ready to Lose Weight?

One reason why even the best diets fail is because people often embark on a weight-loss program before they are truly ready to. Over the years, I've seen many clients who have really wanted to lose weight, but they were not prepared to make the personal commitment necessary to make it happen. Change isn't always easy. Losing weight requires mental and physical energy, dedication, and a willingness to work through the lapses. There are many reasons why people who are highly motivated and well intentioned aren't ready to commit to the process. Buying or selling a home, work stress, marital problems, a death in the family, and financial worries can all be major distractions. That's why I ask every new client I see, "Is the time right?"

To be successful, weight loss must be among your highest priorities. Getting ready to lose weight is crucial to success. To help you prepare yourself for the No-Fail Diet and boost your chance of success, ask yourself the following questions. Your answers will highlight any impediments you have so that you can take steps to overcome them. There is never going to be a perfect time when all conditions are ideal for losing weight. But by understanding what your obstacles might be, you'll increase your chances of losing weight and not gaining it back.

- *How fed up are you with your weight?* If your weight affects your daily life—you don't have enough energy to play with the kids, your back and knees are always hurting, you decline social invitations because your clothes don't fit, you feel self-conscious and lack confidence at work—you're probably ready to make a change.

- *Is now the right time for you?* Even if you are really fed up, you may face obstacles that will make losing weight difficult. Do you face any background obstacles or major stressors that will prevent you from focusing on losing weight? If you do, give yourself a chance to work through them before you start.

- *Do you want to lose weight for yourself or for someone else?* If you want to lose weight because a family member or friend has been nagging you to do so, you're more likely to gain it back. You stand a far better chance of keeping your weight off for good if you want to lose it for yourself. That is, if you want to lose weight because *you* want to look and feel better and have more confidence, you'll be more likely to succeed. You need to do this for yourself and no one else.

- *How long-term is your commitment?* Can you envision eating healthfully and exercising a year from now? Or do you view losing weight as a short-term project that ends once you hit your weight goal? Do you see yourself getting back on track if you go off your plan or miss a workout? If you believe that maintaining a healthy weight is a lifelong commitment and you're motivated to make permanent changes to your lifestyle, you're ready to take action.

- *Do you have friends, family members, or co-workers who will support you in your diet?* You are more likely to stay motivated if you have encouragement along the way. Support comes in many forms—a family commitment to eat healthier, a workout buddy, or simply a friend to talk to. If you don't have someone to be your cheerleader, would you consider joining a weight-loss group or starting one? Sometimes friends and family members can unknowingly sabotage your weight-loss efforts by offering you foods that are off your plan or pressuring you to eat second helpings. Are you prepared to ask them to support you by keeping temptation at bay?

- *Have you resolved any eating disorders or other emotional issues that would get in the way of achieving a healthy weight?* If you binge, use laxatives, or induce vomiting after eating, would you consider seeing a therapist or eating-disorder specialist?

Why the No-Fail Diet?

If you're ready to begin your weight-loss journey, you're ready to start the No-Fail Diet. I told you earlier that fad diets promise "something different," some foolproof plan that will work where other diets have failed. The No-Fail Diet is *not* a fad diet. In fact, it's far from it. And it will work if you want it to. Here's why the No-Fail Diet will help you lose weight and maintain that weight loss.

The No-Fail Diet is nutritionally balanced. Unlike many fad diets, the No-Fail Diet does not exclude entire food groups. You are allowed to eat fruit, whole-grain foods, and dairy products—all those foods with carbohydrates. (However, I will encourage you to choose only the healthiest carbohydrate foods.) By eating a wide variety of healthy foods each day, your body will get all the nutrients it needs. Having said that, sometimes it is not possible to get what you need from foods alone, even if you do eat a balanced diet. To help you meet your daily vitamin and mineral requirements, I give age-specific intake recommendations for key nutrients such as calcium and vitamin D, and guidelines for choosing a supplement if needed.

The No-Fail Diet emphasizes weight maintenance. Successful weight loss means permanent weight loss. That's why I have devoted an entire section of this book to weight maintenance. The No-Fail Diet helps you adjust your food intake once you reach your weight goal. And very importantly, it will teach you lifelong skills to help you stay within your target weight range in the years to come. (Actually,

I think you'll find that is quite easy to do once you realize that losing excess weight and maintaining your new weight are pretty much the same thing.)

The No-Fail Diet is easy to follow because it fits into real life. I don't expect you to live like a hermit while losing weight. That's why you'll be able to stick with my plan. If you enjoy eating in restaurants, no problem: I'll show you how to follow the No-Fail Diet when dining out, even at fast-food courts. And you can include in your plan a favourite dessert or a glass of wine—just not every day. Too busy to cook from scratch? Again, not a problem. The No-Fail Diet gives you plenty of fast and incredibly simple meal ideas—short recipes that can be whipped up in no time with relatively few ingredients. You'll also find recommendations for healthy convenience-food choices at the grocery store. And what about the 2-week vacation you're dreading because you're afraid you'll gain weight? Vacations are allowed. I won't expect you to lose weight, but I will give you some pointers to help you maintain your weight while travelling. An extended trip might slow down your progress, but it won't prevent you from reaching your goal.

The No-Fail Diet focuses on your long-term health. The plan includes foods that keep you healthy. You'll learn how to incorporate foods that help keep blood cholesterol and blood pressure numbers in check, foods that help reduce the risk of developing type 2 diabetes, and foods that help keep our bones strong and minds sharp as we age. At the same time, you'll learn what foods and beverages you need to limit—foods that scientific studies have linked to certain health problems.

The No-Fail Diet does not guarantee quick, dramatic, miraculous results. Sure you can lose 10 pounds in 10 days if you eat nothing but cabbage soup or grapefruit. But that's a short-term fix to a problem that requires a permanent solution. The No-Fail Diet will help you lose weight at a safe rate—about 2 pounds (1 kg) per week. That way you know you're losing body fat, not muscle. When you lose weight too quickly by following a diet that's too low in calories, you end up losing muscle tissue, which causes your metabolism (the speed at which your body burns calories) to slow down. When your metabolism becomes sluggish, it's harder to continue losing weight and, to many people's dismay, much easier to gain it back. Perhaps you've experienced this rebound weight gain yourself after following a crash diet.

The No-Fail Diet does not reject the prevailing wisdom of doctors, dietitians, and nutrition scientists. As a registered dietitian in private practice for close to 20 years, I have seen plenty of fad diets come and go. Many claimed that our prevailing views of weight loss are misguided and offered an unconventional solution. Some downright rejected the wisdom of doctors, dietitians, and nutrition scientists. It's easy to fall for a too-good-to-be-true formula if you're a frustrated yo-yo dieter.

The No-Fail Diet is different. My plan is based on current scientific understanding of what it takes to lose weight and keep it off. There are no gimmicks; just sound, practical advice that—based on many years of experience—I know works. How much you weigh is all about energy balance: calories out versus calories in. In order to lose weight, the calories you burn (calories out) must exceed the calories you eat (calories in). This energy balance equation has been used for years to help people lose weight. Let's face it: Giving up starchy foods, fruit, and dairy on a low-carb diet will drastically reduce one's calorie intake. Most experts agree that the fat loss from these diets is the result of eating fewer calories, not from some magical effect a lower intake of carbohydrates has on our bodies' chemicals or hormones.

The No-Fail Diet's Four Keys to Success

The No-Fail Diet is based on four principles, principles that I've used repeatedly over the years to help my clients permanently lose weight. These four factors are critical to help you feel satisfied and full longer after eating, feel energized during the day, and keep you motivated during your weight-loss journey. They've worked for thousands of my clients, and I know they will work for you, too.

1. The Timing Factor

On the No-Fail Diet, you must eat every 3 to 4 hours during the day (between 6 A.M. and 7 P.M.). That means you must eat three meals plus one or two snacks, depending on your schedule. If your meals are to be eaten more than 4 hours apart, you must plan to have a small snack to prevent you from becoming too hungry. We all know what happens when we get too hungry—we grab whatever is handy to fill the gap (usually something junky) or we overeat at the next meal.

Think about how you feel when you get home from work at the end of a stressful day. Imagine you have not eaten since noon, when you quickly wolfed down a sandwich. If you're like most of my clients, you're feeling tired, irritable, and very hungry. Then the snacking starts—crackers, a piece of cheese, maybe a cookie or two. You may even sneak a few tastings while preparing dinner. Sound familiar? By the time you actually sit down to your evening meal, you may have easily eaten an entire meal's worth of calories.

Now think about how you might feel had you eaten a snack mid-afternoon. I am willing to bet you would walk in the door with your appetite under control. You would feel calmer, less irritable, and ready to tackle dinner preparation without first raiding the cupboards for a snack. And more than likely, you would find it easier to eat smaller portions at dinner.

Eating at regular intervals does more than curb your appetite and prevent overeating. While that's critical to sticking with the No-Fail Diet, eating every 3 to 4 hours also fuels your body, preparing it for the physical challenges of the day. If you work out at lunch time, you'll need to eat a late-morning snack to provide energy to your muscles. If you have a little fuel in your system, you'll be able to work out harder, recover faster, and get better results. Eating at regular intervals during the day also fuels your brain cells, enhancing your short-term memory and ability to concentrate.

The timing factor starts with breakfast. You must eat breakfast every day: Skipping is not allowed. Eating breakfast helps kick-start your metabolism and prevents you from becoming too hungry before lunch, making you more likely to make reasonable lunch choices.

People who eat breakfast on a regular basis are more likely to have a structured eating plan throughout the day and are less likely to snack on empty calorie foods. Don't worry if you don't like eating breakfast: Your body will adjust in short time to eating a morning meal.

One of my clients, Rachel, came to see me to lose 25 pounds. She never ate breakfast and often skipped lunch. She typically came home from work, nibbled on some cheese, and then ate a balanced dinner with her husband. She complained that she didn't feel satisfied after dinner and usually snacked while watching television. I designed a meal plan for Rachel that included breakfast, lunch, afternoon snack, and dinner. She stuck with it and, sure enough, after three months of following my plan, she reached her goal of losing 25 pounds. What's more, her after-dinner food cravings for chocolate disappeared. I continue to see Rachel to help her maintain her new weight. She firmly believes the key to her weight-loss success is eating breakfast.

Rachel's story is common. People who skip meals, especially breakfast, and don't eat midday snacks say they don't feel satisfied even after a healthy dinner. They crave foods in the evening and end up back-loading the bulk of their day's calories at the end the day, a time when their bodies aren't as efficient at burning off those calories. Eating smaller meals during the day instead of one or two big ones later in the day helps reduce food cravings and triggers the body to burn fuel more efficiently. Gorging on one or two calorie-laden meals makes it easier for your body to store energy as fat.

Even scientists agree that starting your day with a morning meal helps you eat less during the day. Researchers from the University of Texas studied almost 900 men and women to learn how meal timing influenced their day's calorie intake. Like my client Rachel, the researchers found that calories consumed in the morning helped curb appetite and reduce the amount of food eaten for the remainder of the day. But when calories were eaten later in the day, participants lacked the same feeling of fullness (satiety), and this led to snacking— and a higher intake of calories for the day.[1]

Everyone's schedule is different, so there isn't one eating timetable that's ideal for everyone. How you apply the timing factor will depend on your schedule. Your weekend eating schedule may differ from your weekday schedule, and that's okay. Just remember, the goal is to eat every 3 to 4 hours during the day (the clock stops at dinner—that means no evening snacking). Listen to your body and use common sense when deciding what times to eat during the day. Snacks should not be eaten too close to meal times; schedule snacks 2 to 3 hours apart from meals.

Here are a few examples of eating schedules that will help you feel energized and satiated while losing weight on the No-Fail Diet. Which one most closely matches your day?

Breakfast:	7:00–7:30 a.m.	Breakfast:	8:00–8:30 a.m.
Morning snack:	10:00–10:30 a.m.	Morning snack:	Not needed
Lunch:	Noon–1:00 p.m.	Lunch:	Noon–1:00 p.m.
Afternoon snack:	3:00–4:00 p.m.	Afternoon snack:	3:00–3:30 p.m.
Dinner:	7:00–7:30 p.m.	Dinner:	6:00–6:30 p.m.
Breakfast:	6:00–6:30 a.m.	Breakfast:	6:30–7:00 a.m.
Morning snack:	9:00–9:30 a.m.	Morning snack:	9:30–10:30 a.m.
Lunch:	Noon–1:00 p.m.	Lunch:	1:00–2:00 p.m.
Afternoon snack:	3:00–4:00 p.m.	Afternoon snack:	3:30–4:00 p.m.
Dinner:	6:30–7:30 p.m.	Dinner:	6:30–7:30 p.m.

There's one more rule in the timing factor: *You must finish eating dinner by 8 p.m.* While there is no scientific evidence that eating late can make you gain weight, my clinical experience tells me that it does. In my private practice, clients who make a habit of eating their main meal late in the evening have more difficulty controlling their weight. When they break this habit and eat dinner earlier, losing weight becomes easier. There is research to support this observation too. Researchers from France revealed that the body burns more calories digesting a meal in the morning and afternoon than it does in the evening meal.[2]

And let's not forget that most of us are less active in the evening. A meal eaten in the middle of the day is usually followed by several hours of activity. Our body is busy using up these calories and nutrients to fuel our day's activities. But most of us are sedentary after eating dinner, watching television, reading, or sleeping. Eating large meals late in the evening means that more of the calories you consume will be stored as body fat.

I realize you can't always make it home in time to finish eating dinner by 8 P.M. For those nights when you walk in the door late, make a compromise. Tell yourself it's too late to eat a full dinner. Instead have a mini meal or snack—a bowl of soup, a half sandwich, yogurt with fruit, or a small salad with 3 ounces (90 g) of chicken breast. Weekends are another story. When you're entertaining guests, or dining out, you're often eating after 8 P.M. That's okay, too. A late meal once a week certainly isn't going to affect your ability to lose weight. They key is to make it an exception rather than the rule.

2. The Protein Factor

On the No-Fail Diet, you must eat a source of protein with every meal and snack. Dietary protein plays an important role in helping you control how much food you eat during the day. Compared with carbohydrate and fat, protein keeps you feeling full longer after eating a meal, for the entire day, and even over the longer term. That's because high-protein foods such as chicken, fish, meat, legumes, and yogurt slow the movement of food from your stomach. Slower stomach emptying means you'll feel satisfied longer. Eating a meal or snack that includes a source of protein also has a smooth, steady effect on your blood sugar. When you eat a meal that includes only rapidly digested carbohydrates, such as white bread or a cereal bar, your blood sugar rises and falls quickly, bringing on hunger pangs. And here's another bonus: Your body burns up more calories to digest protein than it does to break down carbohydrate and fat.

Protein-rich foods supply the body with amino acids, compounds that are used to make hormones, antibodies, enzymes, and haemoglobin, which carries oxygen in your blood. In the body, protein is also used to keep your muscles, bones, skin, and hair healthy. We all need a certain amount of protein each day to stay healthy. If you're sedentary, you need roughly one-third of a gram of protein per pound (0.8 grams of protein per kilogram) of body weight each day to keep your tissues from breaking down. If you play sports or participate in endurance or strength training, you need a little more. You'll have no problem meeting your daily protein needs on the No-Fail Diet.

You certainly don't need to eat protein to the exclusion of everything else. In fact, research suggests that overloading on protein foods can weaken your bones.[3] The No-Fail Diet meal plan has been carefully designed to balance quality proteins with healthy carbohydrates and fat at every meal and most snacks. What do I consider a quality protein food? It's one that's low in cholesterol-raising saturated fat and packed with plenty of nutrients such as iron, zinc, calcium, and magnesium. (You'll read more about the top foods to pick in Chapter 3.) Here's a list of protein-rich foods that add that fullness factor to meals and snacks:

lean beef	milk	soy milk	energy bars*
lean pork	latte	soybeans	
chicken	yogurt	kidney beans	
turkey	low-fat cheese	black beans	
fish	eggs, whole	chickpeas	
shellfish	egg whites	lentils	
		nuts	

* I'll tell you what to look for when buying energy bars in Chapter 4.

3. The Portion-Size Factor

On the No-Fail Diet, you will learn to manage the amount of food you eat by mastering the skills of portion control. Many of my clients tell me they know their portion sizes are too big. They snack out of economy-size bags of pretzels, eat too much pasta at dinner, or polish off a steak meant to serve two people, and often admit to going back for seconds. They recognize that a lack of portion control is a big reason why they're overweight. But some clients *don't* realize they're eating too much and wonder why they can't lose weight. A good example is Carol, who came to see me to take off 20 pounds. She told me she ate only healthy foods and was stumped why her weight wasn't budging. She told me she didn't eat any fast food, sweets, or high-fat snacks. Her typical breakfast was a bowl of whole-grain cereal, fresh berries, and skim milk. She bought her lunch from a popular salad bar, snacked on almonds midday, and often ate fish and steamed vegetables for dinner.

Sounds like a perfect plan for weight loss, right? It wasn't until I asked about her portion sizes that the reason she couldn't lose weight became evident. When I showed her food models and asked her to compare her intake to the models, I learned that Carol ate 2 cups (500 ml) of whole-grain cereal at breakfast (twice as much as she needed). She added too many high-fat ingredients to her salad at lunch (3 oz/90 g cheese, 3 tbsp/50 ml sunflower seeds, half an avocado, and plenty of dressing). Her afternoon snack consisted of a few handfuls of almonds (about 450 calories), and her usual fish portion measured a good 8 ounces (240 g). Carol is a classic case of someone who eats the right foods in portions that are just too big.

Scaling down on portions is key to losing weight. Today, food portions have gotten so incredibly huge at restaurants and coffee shops that many people have lost the ability to judge how much food is too much. They might even have trouble recognizing a normal portion. Even packaged foods in the grocery store have steadily grown in size since the 1960s. Thanks to inflated portion sizes, you might eat more than you think. Consider these facts:

- Bagels used to be 2 to 3 ounces (60 to 90 g), or 200 calories. Today they're 5 to 6 ounces (150 to 180 g) and have as many as 400 calories. If you eat a 5 ounce (150 g) bagel from Tim Hortons or Starbucks, you'll be consuming the carbohydrate equivalent of five slices of bread or 15 cups (3.75 litres) of air-popped popcorn.

- Muffins used to be 1 1/2 ounces (45 g) and 205 calories. Now they average almost 5 ounces (150 g) and 400 calories.

- One cup (250 ml) of cooked pasta used to be a typical restaurant serving. Now some restaurants serve 3 to 4 cups (750 to 1000 ml) of pasta, delivering as many as 800 calories without the sauce.

- Twenty years ago, soft drinks were sold in small 6 1/2 ounce (192 ml) bottles, which provided 74 calories and about

4 teaspoons (20 ml) worth of sugar. Today, single servings are three times bigger. Soft drinks are now sold in 20 ounce (591 ml) bottles, a portion that serves up 230 calories to your waistline (almost 14 tsp/70 ml of sugar).

It's easy to see that portion size can influence how many calories you eat. Larger portions of food have more calories, which can lead to weight gain if you don't burn them off with exercise. Several studies have shown that serving older kids and adults larger food portions of snacks and meals leads to significant increases in calorie intake. What's more, despite increases in food intake, people presented with large portions generally don't report increased levels of fullness, suggesting that our body's hunger and satiety signals are ignored when we eat supersize portions.

What's a Serving?

A *portion size* is simply the amount of food you choose to eat at one sitting, whether it's from a restaurant, from a package, or from your own kitchen. *A serving size,* on the other hand, isn't what you just happen to put on your plate. It's a specific amount of food defined by Canada's Food Guide, nutrition labels, some cookbooks, and many diet plans. It's serving sizes that you need to pay attention to. The No-Fail Diet defines standard serving sizes and tells you how many servings of foods to eat based on your calorie and nutrient needs. You just need to adjust your current portion sizes so they match your recommended servings on the No-Fail Diet. (You'll find the list of food and standard serving sizes in Chapter 4.)

Learning portion control isn't as difficult as you may think. All you have to do is train yourself to be able to eyeball appropriate serving sizes of your favourite foods. The No-Fail Diet will show you three ways to assess the portion size of the foods you eat. I recommend you try all three of these methods to find the one that works best for you. Once you get into the habit of monitoring your portions, it will be second nature.

1. Measure Your Food. The best way to figure out how much you're eating is to measure it. *For the first 2 weeks on the No-Fail Diet, measure* *your foods in a measuring cup or with measuring spoons.* You'll need to learn what 1 cup (250 ml) of breakfast cereal, 1 cup (250 ml) of cooked pasta, and 3 ounces (90 g) of cooked chicken look like in your bowl or on your plate. You'll need to learn what 4 teaspoons (20 ml) of salad dressing looks like drizzled over your salad. After 2 weeks, you'll become an expert at knowing what an appropriate portion size is just by sight—you won't need to measure. But because portion sizes can easily creep up over time, I recommend that you refresh your memory every so often by measuring your foods.

You also need to start reading nutrition labels on food packages to become familiar with serving sizes of your favourite brands of cereal, crackers, soup, and even salad dressing. The numbers on the Nutrition Facts box—the calories, grams of fat, protein, sugar, fibre, and so on—apply to 1 serving of the food. If you eat 2 servings, double the numbers. You might be surprised to learn that 1 serving is much less than what you're used to eating.

2. Eyeball Your Portions. If measuring your food makes you crazy, eyeball your foods to make sure you're eating a proper serving size. It's easy to translate serving-size information into something visual that's easy to remember. Use the following list to compare serving sizes of particular foods with familiar objects:

1 serving of ...	Looks like ...
Bagel, 1/2	A hockey puck
Butter, margarine, 1 tsp (5 ml)	The tip of your thumb or a dice
Cheese, 1 1/2 oz (45 g)	Three dominos
Fish, meat, chicken, 3 oz (90 g)	A deck of playing cards
Fish, thin fillet, baked/grilled, 3 oz (90 g)	A chequebook
Fruit, 1 medium	A baseball
Muffin, 1 small	A large egg
Pancake, 1	A CD
Pasta or rice, cooked, 1/2 cup (125 ml)	Half a baseball, or an ice cream scoop
Peanut butter, 2 tbsp (25 ml)	A ping-pong ball
Potato, baked, 1 small	A computer mouse
Salad greens, 1 cup (250 ml)	A baseball
Vegetables, cooked, 1/2 cup (125 ml)	Half a baseball, or a small fist

3. The Plate Model. This is a good method to use if you're eating a buffet-style meal, but you can use it for any type of meal. It requires that you look at your plate and think about the proportion of food on it and the portion sizes you're eating. Take a look at your dinner plate. Is half of it covered by a slab of meat? Is it overflowing with spaghetti and meat sauce? Here's how the plate model helps you eat appropriate portion sizes: Divide your dinner plate into four sections, or quarters. Fill one quarter with your protein food—meat, chicken, fish, or tofu. Fill another quarter with starchy foods such as rice, pasta, potato, or quinoa. The remaining half of your plate is to be filled with cooked vegetables and salad greens.

Courtesy of iDesign® Inc.

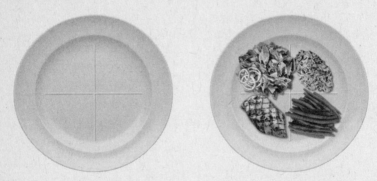

Some people find it easier to visualize their plate as a clock, filling the 12 to 6 slot with veggies, the 6 to 9 slot with starchy foods, and the 9 to 12 slot with protein.

Portion Control Tips

Even if you do measure out your food portions, overcoming the temptation to overeat can be challenging if your appetite is accustomed to eating more food than you need. Here are a few strategies to help you pare down your portions, whether you're eating at home, in a restaurant, or even at the movies.

- Buy small packages of food. Economy-size boxes of cookies and snack foods encourage overeating. If you shop in bulk, break jumbo-size packages into smaller, individual portions as soon as you get home.

- Read the Nutrition Facts box on the food package. Don't assume that large food packages or drink containers yield only 1 serving. Check to see how many servings one package contains.

- Don't snack directly from the package. Whether you snack on dried fruit, popcorn, or baked tortilla chips, measure out 1 serving and put it on a plate or in a small bowl. Trust me: You'll end up eating less.

- Add fruit and vegetables to your meals. Fruits and veggies contain fibre and water; they add volume to meals and can help you feel satisfied on fewer calories.

- Use a smaller plate. Instead of filling a dinner plate, serve your meal on a luncheon-size plate. The plate will look full and you'll end up eating less. Many of my clients have told me that serving their dinner on a luncheon-size plate really helped them lose weight. One client, Sarah, told me during a follow-up visit that she had been following this strategy for the past 2 months. The result was a 10-pound weight loss. If you don't have luncheon-size plates, I recommend that you use dinner plates that measure no more than 9 inches (22 cm) in diameter.

- Ask for smaller portions when dining out. Split an entree with a friend, or order two appetizers instead of an entree. At fast-food outlets avoid "extra value," "king size," or "biggie" meals.

- Slow your pace. After every bite, put down your knife and fork and chew your food thoroughly. It takes about 20 minutes for your brain to register you've had enough to eat. If you eat too quickly, you're more likely to overeat.

- Avoid distractions while eating, such as watching television or reading. You need to pay attention to the fact you're eating to help you feel satisfied. Savour every bite.

4. The Tracking Factor

On the No-Fail Diet, you will monitor your progress to enhance your weight-loss success. Self-monitoring is a powerful tool that helps you succeed at losing weight—and keeping it off. Monitoring and tracking your food intake, daily exercise, body measurements, weight, and even the emotions you experience provides you with immediate feedback. Only by tracking can you know how well you're doing, or if you need to make a few changes to improve your rate of weight loss. On the No-Fail Diet, tracking your progress will involve keeping tabs on your food intake, physical activity, and your body measurements. Here are the tools you'll need.

1. A Food Journal

One of the most important tools in successful weight loss is a food journal. A food journal will provide awareness of your eating habits and keep you focused on and committed to your goals. It will highlight, in black and white, the foods you are eating and your portion sizes. It will also reveal the healthy foods you might not be eating enough of. Filling out a food journal will make you think twice about eating a second helping at dinner or sneaking a few bites from your child's plate. Writing down what you eat will help you avoid mindless eating (the nibbles you don't pay attention to and easily forget), uncover emotional eating patterns, identify overeating triggers, and, of course, keep track of your daily food servings.

You'll find a Daily Food and Activity Tracker in Appendix 1. I suggest you photocopy these pages before you start filling them in so that you have plenty of extras. You can carry your Food and Activity Tracker with you during the day. Or if you prefer, create your own food journal on a pad of paper or in a bound notebook. Write down the time of day you ate, the foods you ate, and your portion sizes. On the Food and Activity Tracker you'll also be able to tally your total intake of food group servings for the day and compare it to your No-Fail Diet meal plan. For example, if you record that you ate 3 ounces (90 g) of turkey in your sandwich, that counts as 3 Protein Food servings. If you eat 1 cup (250 ml) of cooked pasta at dinner, that counts as 2 Starchy Food servings. (You'll learn about the food groups and serving sizes in Chapter 4.) Record your food intake after each meal. Don't wait until the end of the day to complete your food journal because you're likely to forget a few foods.

I also encourage you to think about your hunger level prior to eating and how full you felt after eating. Listening to your body can help prevent you from eating too many calories. Use the following scale to assess how you feel before you eat, halfway through a meal, and after you finish eating. Your goal is to stop eating when you reach level 5 on the hunger scale.

Hunger Scale

Level	How Hungry You Feel
1	You feel starving. You can't concentrate because your stomach feels so empty. You need food now!
2	You feel hungry and know that your stomach needs food, but you could wait a few minutes before eating.
3	You feel a slightly hungry. You could eat something, but you couldn't eat a large meal.
4	Your hunger has almost disappeared. You could eat another bite.
5	You are no longer hungry. You feel satisfied but not full.
6	You feel slightly full.
7	You feel overly full and uncomfortable. Your waistband is noticeably tighter.
8	You feel stuffed, bloated, even nauseous. Some people call this the "Thanksgiving Day full."

Also consider any overriding emotions that are present when you eat. Did you eat because you were bored? Stressed? Depressed? Distracted? Uncovering emotions that trigger eating is important for your long-term success at losing weight and preventing weight regain.

Many of my clients use their food journals not only to track their intake but also to plan their meals in advance. They write down the foods and portion sizes they will eat *one day in advance*. Planning ahead helps you be prepared for the next day. For instance, if you know that the better part of tomorrow is going to be spent running errands, you can plan in advance where you will stop for lunch and what you will order. You'll be able to foresee the need to pack portable snacks with you. Writing your food journal one day in advance also removes the stress of last-minute meal planning. You will know what you're going to prepare for tomorrow's dinner and as a result, you can make sure you have all the ingredients handy.

There's scientific evidence that taking a daily inventory of what you eat, how much you eat, and when you eat can help you control your weight. A 2005 study published in the *New England Journal of Medicine* found that among people who took a prescription weight-loss medication and underwent lifestyle-modification counselling, those who frequently recorded their daily food intake lost more weight than those who did so less often.[4]

And there's more research to show that food journals work. The National Weight Control Registry is a U.S. database of over 5000 people who have maintained at least a 30-pound (13.5 kg) weight loss for a minimum of 1 year. Researchers have learned that one of the key habits of these highly successful dieters is keeping a food journal. One-half of all participants say they record their daily food intake and workouts.[5]

2. *Physical Activity Tracker*

Keeping tabs on your daily exercise will help you track your fitness progress, set goals for improvement, and identify the activities you like best. There's no need to keep a separate journal for your daily exercise. I've made it easy for you to monitor your daily physical activity on the Food and Activity Tracker. In the Daily Activity section, write down the type of exercise you do each day and how long you spend doing it. Include daily walking, biking, and gardening, as well as any fitness classes and workouts at the gym. You'll also find a 12-Week Fitness Tracker in Appendix 1 that will help you monitor your progress on the No-Fail 12-Week Fitness Program (discussed in Chapter 5).

3. Body Measurement Tracker

When you're losing weight, it's incredibly motivating to watch your measurements get smaller. Seeing the results of your efforts provides impetus to keep going. On the No-Fail Diet, I ask you to keep track of the following:

Your weight—once per week. Pick the same day of the week, preferably first thing in the morning when you're naturally your lightest (we tend to gain a little water weight during the day), to weigh yourself. If you weigh-in at the gym, do this before you workout, not after. During exercise, you lose weight from sweating. For every pound you lose from sweating, you need to drink 2 cups (500 ml) of water to replace your fluid loss.

Don't get into the bad habit of weighing yourself every day. That's a mistake. It's normal for your weight to fluctuate daily from fluid retention, even a bout of constipation. You won't see progress if you weigh-in daily, so don't set yourself up for frustration and disappointment.

If you're starting a new exercise program, or ramping up your existing one, keep in mind that the scale might not show your results right away. That's because muscle weighs more than body fat. So if you're building a little muscle and losing fat at the same time, the numbers on the scale might move more slowly than you'd expect during the first few weeks on your new workout regime. But there's no need to worry—you will see results. Just be patient. This is the reason why it's so important to keep track of your body measurements too. Even if the scale is slow to move, you'll be thrilled to see your waistline shrink.

Your body measurements—when you start the No-Fail Diet and once per month thereafter. You'll need a measuring tape to track the following (with the exception of body mass index):

- *Body mass index (BMI):* You'll learn how to calculate this number and what it means in the next section.

- *Waist:* Without holding the tape too tightly or too loosely, measure your waist circumference. Your waist is the narrowest part of your trunk, about 1 inch (2.5 cm) above your belly button.

- *Hips:* Standing with your heels together, measure your hips around the fullest part of your buttocks.

- *Waist-to-hip ratio (WHR):* This is your waist measurement divided by your hip measurement. For example, if you have a 35 inch waist and 46 inch hips, your WHR is 0.76 (35 ÷ 46 = 0.76). For women, WHR should be 0.8 or less; for men 0.95 or less. If your WHR is higher, you're at increased health risk because you carry more fat around your middle (abdominal fat).

- *Chest/bust:* Take your measurement around the fullest part of your chest.

You can keep track of all your measurements with the 12-Week Body Measurement Tracker on page 342 in Appendix 1. There are other numbers you might want to track, too. Some of my clients like to keep track of their clothing size—pant size, suit size, dress size, and so on. If you have access to fitness testing, you might want to keep track of your body fat percentage (once every 3 months). It also might be important for you to monitor certain health measurements, such as your blood pressure or blood cholesterol numbers.

Setting Your Personal Weight Goal

Now that you have a good understanding of how the four factors of the No-Fail Diet will help you succeed at losing weight, it's time for you to decide on your weight goal. How much weight do you want to lose? Or rather, how much weight do you need to lose to feel healthier, happier, and more energetic?

Before you answer that question, it's important to assess your current weight in terms of health. (Perhaps you don't need to lose as much weight as you think you do.) You can then determine what a healthy weight is for you. Although there is some debate over what constitutes a healthy weight, I believe that a healthy weight is based on the ratio of your weight to height. This ratio is called the body mass index (BMI). Many studies have found that a BMI above 25 increases the risk of dying early from heart disease and certain cancers and that a BMI above 30 dramatically increases the risk.

Your weight is considered to be healthy if your BMI is between 20 and 25 (some research suggests the healthiest weight corresponds to a BMI between 18.5 and 22). Overweight is defined by a BMI of 25 to 29.9, and obesity is defined as a BMI above 30. Here's how to calculate your BMI (you'll need a pencil and calculator):

1.	Determine your body weight in kilograms (divide weight in pounds by 2.2) Your weight in kilograms =
2.	Determine your height in centimetres (multiply height in inches by 2.54) Your height in centimetres =
3.	Determine your height in metres (divide height in centimetres by 100) Your height in metres =
4.	Square your height in metres (multiply height in metres by height in metres) Your height in metres^2 =
5.	Now, calculate your BMI (divide weight in kilograms by height in metres^2) Your BMI =

If your BMI is over 25, determine what you need to weigh in order to have a healthy BMI. In other words, what do you need to weigh to achieve a BMI of 25? That's a great weight to set your personal weight goal at. Once you've achieved that weight by following the No-Fail Diet, you can decide if it's realistic to strive for a lower BMI. Keep in mind, though, that losing as little as 5% to 10% of your current body weight can still lead to important improvements in weight-related health conditions such as high blood pressure, high blood cholesterol, and elevated blood sugar.

If you're athletic or have a muscular build, your BMI might be a little higher than you would expect. That's because muscle and bone weigh more than fat. So if you are a muscular person, be realistic when it comes to choosing a weight goal based on BMI. It's probably not realistic to achieve a BMI in the low 20s. And that's fine.

What if your current weight falls within the healthy BMI zone of 20 to 25? Does that mean you don't need to lose weight? No, it doesn't. You'll notice that the healthy BMI zone encompasses quite a wide weight range. For example, my BMI is in the healthy range if I weigh between 130 to 160 pounds. Now, if I weighed 160 pounds, my BMI would be 25, but I wouldn't fit into my clothes. And I wouldn't be too pleased about that. What I'm saying is that just because your BMI is 24 or 25, this doesn't mean you aren't carrying around an extra 10 to 15 pounds of body fat. Those extra pounds might not be influencing your health, but they very well could be impacting your self-esteem.

When deciding on your weight goal, you also need to consider your weight history over the past 10 to 20 years. That's because how much weight you've gained since your mid-20s strongly influences your chances of developing certain health problems, including diabetes, heart disease, gallstones, and sleep apnea. If you haven't gained more than 10 pounds since you were 21, that's great. Work on keeping your weight steady. If you decide to tackle that extra weight that has crept on since college, that's great, too. This book will help you do that.

Reviewing your personal weight history also helps you maintain perspective when choosing your weight goal. You need to be realistic when determining how much weight you want to lose. Being realistic means considering your lifestyle and what changes you're willing to make. There's no sense in setting your sights on a weight that's impossible to achieve because your current lifestyle just won't permit it. Susan's story is a perfect example of this point.

When I first met with Susan, she told me that she wanted to get back to the 118 pounds she weighed in her early 20s, a time when she was single and able to work out at the gym 5 days a week. For Susan, this meant losing 40 pounds. Never mind that at the age of 49, Susan's metabolism has slowed down a little over the past 25 years. More importantly, she's now a busy mother of three children, with a demanding job that frequently involves dining out with clients. As for exercise, she can only manage to squeeze three brisk 30-minute walks into her hectic week's schedule—a far cry from the daily aerobic classes she once did.

When I told Susan what lifestyle changes she would need to make in order to return to 118 pounds, she agreed that they just weren't realistic. Her job was not going to change; she had to deal with the fact that dining out was a big part of her life. And with three active kids, she couldn't spend hours at the gym like she used to. We agreed, however, that it was realistic for her to lose 30 pounds and achieve a weight of 128 pounds. This was a weight that, given her current lifestyle, she would be able to maintain. Once Susan realized this, she was very pleased and excited with her new goal.

The point I am making is that you need to be realistic, not idealistic, about your weight. Don't get me wrong. I've helped many clients achieve the weights they were at in their early 20s. But sometimes it's just not practical. If your expectations are unrealistic, you will disappoint yourself and give up. The following questions, along with your BMI calculations, will help you determine what weight is right for you:

1. What is your current weight? _____

   How long have you been at this weight? _____

2. What did you weigh: 1 year ago? _____ 5 years ago? _____

   10 years ago? _____ 20 years ago (if applicable)? _____

3. At what weight did you feel your best (you felt healthy, energetic, and had high self-esteem)? _____

4. If there were no obstacles in your life, what would you like to weigh? _____

   (This is your ideal weight goal.)

5. If you were to be realistic about your lifestyle, what weight would you be satisfied to achieve and maintain? (This is your realistic weight goal; for some of you it might be the same as your idealistic weight goal.) _____

   What will your body mass index (BMI) be at this weight? _____

6. Express your weight goal as a weight range (e.g., 130 to 135 lbs/ 59 to 61 kg). It's not realistic to always maintain one number on the scale. You need to allow a little leeway for natural day-to-day

weight fluctuations, not to mention a few pounds you might gain on a holiday. Choose a weight with a 3 to 5 pound (1.5 to 2.5 kg) range that you will be comfortable staying within. This is called your buffer zone—the weight range that you will always maintain.

My realistic buffer zone is _____ lbs/kg to _____ lbs/kg.

7. How much weight do you need to lose to achieve this goal?
   _____

Staying Motivated on the No-Fail Diet— Thinking Right

Now that you've determined your weight goal, you're almost ready to begin the No-Fail Diet. Getting ready to lose weight also requires examining your mindset and, if necessary, adopting new attitudes. An important predictor of weight-loss success is how you think. You may not realize it, but your thoughts can help you achieve your goals, or they can sabotage your efforts. An unhealthy mindset can undermine the very behaviours you're trying so hard to change.

Pretend you're already at the weight you'd like to be. This may sound strange, but thinking like a thinner person can help you develop a positive image of yourself. By building an image of yourself at your goal weight, you'll boost your self-confidence and self-image. There's no need to wait to do this until you reach your weight goal. Bolstering your self-esteem right now will help you succeed at losing weight.

Acting in the way you will feel and think when you're thinner will help your goals come true. So how can you think like a thinner person? Some people find it helps to visualize themselves as slimmer. They hang a favourite outfit they want to fit into again where they'll see it every day, or they tack an old photograph of themselves at a healthy weight on the fridge. It also helps to think about how you felt at a lighter weight—how differently you walked, talked, and moved when you were 15, 25, or 40 pounds lighter.

Perhaps you can't remember how you felt when you weighed less. If that's the case, think about how great you *will* feel when you lose your weight and how this will influence how you interact with the people in your life. Think about food in terms of nutrition and fuel rather than as an emotional crutch. Reflect on these feelings every day. Each morning, tell yourself you look great (because you do) and then go out and act on these visions and feelings. You are what you think.

Change your attitude. Believing that you *can* lose weight is a strong predictor of success. Even researchers agree. In a study from the Netherlands, 66 overweight men and women were put on an 8-week low-calorie diet. Before entering the study, all participants were asked about their self-esteem, mental health, eating behaviours, support network, and reasons for being overweight. At the end of the study, the researchers found that those persons who perceived themselves as being able to succeed at losing weight lost significantly more weight than those who were less sure of their ability to stick to the weight-loss program.[6]

To believe in your ability to achieve your goal, you need to get rid of any negative thought patterns you have. One mindset that works against weight loss is all-or-nothing thinking. I sometimes glimpse this thinking pattern in clients who feel they're either "on" or "off" their diets. They pat themselves on the back for being good when they're following their meal plan and getting regular exercise. But the slightest slip will make them feel as though they're being bad. I call this the diet mentality, and it's one that causes people to continuously struggle with their weight.

Adopting behaviours that lead to weight loss is not an all-or-nothing endeavour. You don't have to be perfect to succeed. If you're on track 80% of the time, you'll do just fine. It's perfectly normal to slip up occasionally—we're human after all. One lapse isn't going to ruin all your hard work. The key is getting back on track as soon as you can.

You can maintain your motivation to lose weight by telling yourself every day that you can and will succeed. Banish any negative statements from your head and replace them with positive affirmations.

Instead of saying you *can't* or you *should,* tell yourself out loud that you *can* and you *will.* If you make positive self-talk your mode of operation, you'll notice a difference in your ability to make changes that promote weight loss.

Be assertive. It's important to learn to say no. Whether that means turning down sweets at the office or asking a server to bring your salad dressing on the side, being assertive will get you closer to your goals. Being assertive isn't always easy, especially with family and friends. But you need to remind yourself that weight loss is in your power and nobody else is going to do it for you. It's all up to you. After all, that's who you're doing this for.

Be patient. If you expect to lose your weight overnight you will feel frustrated and disappointed. And disappointment can easily lead to giving up. You need to accept that slow, steady weight loss is the right way to permanently lose weight. Losing weight at a rate of 1 to 2 pounds (0.5 to 1 kg) per week has proved safe, healthy, and effective. People who lose weight slowly tend to keep their weight off over the long term. If you're someone who wants instant gratification, you'd better rethink how you measure your progress. Instead of focusing on the bathroom scale, think about other meaningful changes. Remind yourself about the positive changes you've made to your eating habits, the improvements in your fitness level, the increased amount of energy you feel each day, or the fact that your blood pressure has decreased. There are many benefits to weight loss besides the number on the scale. So be realistic, be patient, and focus on all the positive changes you experience along the way.

Reward your successes. Don't hold off on congratulating yourself until you reach your final weight goal. Every small success deserves a pat on the back. Rewarding yourself as you meet small goals is a way to remind yourself that you can do it. Determine which achievements you will reward. Getting to the gym 4 days this week? Breaking the habit of eating while watching television? Losing 5 pounds? Then plan what your rewards will be—a new CD, a pair of running shoes, a massage or pedicure? You don't need to spend money to reward yourself. Simple luxuries such as soaking in a bubble bath, reading a novel, or watching a movie can also make you feel good about yourself.

2

Getting and Staying Active

You won't lose weight unless you're burning more calories than you're eating. I'm sure it comes as no surprise that exercise plays an important role in weight control by increasing your body's energy output. Exercise burns calories while you're doing it, and it causes your metabolism to stay increased for a period after you finish, allowing you to burn off extra calories. (Your metabolism is the energy you use to keep your body alive—to keep your heart beating, your lungs breathing, and your body temperature regulated. It accounts for 50% to 75% of your daily calorie expenditure.)

You might be thinking that people lose weight all the time without exercise, just by eating less. And that's true. Reducing the amount of food you eat tends to have more of an impact on weight loss than exercise does because it's relatively easy to significantly reduce your daily calorie intake. For instance, if you cut 300 calories each day—simply by giving up those three cookies in the afternoon—you'd save 9000 calories per month, a savings that translates into a 2.5 pound (1 kg) loss on the bathroom scale. To burn off 300 calories through exercise, you'd have to walk the dog briskly for 1 hour or jog for 27 minutes. (These numbers are based on a body weight of 150 lbs/68 kg. A heavier person will expend more calories and lighter people will burn less.) As you can see, you'd have to exercise a lot in order to lose 2.5 pounds (1 kg) each month.

How Exercise Helps You Permanently Lose Weight

No matter how much exercise you do, you won't lose weight if you eat more than you burn. In fact, study after study shows that when people are told to lose weight with diet or exercise, the dieters always lose significantly more weight than the exercisers. While it might be easier to lose weight by making dietary changes alone, compared with only adding exercise, it's the combination of the two that works best.

There are three reasons why the mix of exercise and eating less offers the most effective approach to losing weight. For starters, burning extra calories through exercise allows you to eat a little more food while losing weight. Second, if you eat too few calories and don't exercise, you'll lose weight but you might sacrifice some of your muscle mass. Losing muscle results in a slower metabolism, which makes it difficult to continue losing weight and keeping it off. (The amount of muscle you have is linked to your metabolism; the more muscle you have, the more calories your body burns at rest.) Adding strengthening exercises such as weight training, biking, or spinning classes can help you preserve muscle and boost your metabolism.

There's one more very important reason why you need to add exercise to your weight-loss program. Exercise is crucial for keeping the pounds off once you lose them. The vast majority of people who lose weight without exercising regain their weight. However, research shows that 95% of people who successfully lose weight and keep it off do so by exercising almost daily.[1]

Getting regular physical activity also boosts your self-esteem. My clients who exercise feel good about themselves, and this positive feeling often carries over to their eating habits. There's no question that exercise and eating right are closely linked. Compared with sedentary folks, people who work out on a regular basis are much more likely to make healthy food choices. After all, who wants to sabotage *all that* hard work on the treadmill by eating one lousy doughnut?

Of course, there are many other good reasons why you should get active and stay active. Regular moderate exercise can improve your mood, enhance your body's ability to fight infection, slow down age-related bone loss, and reduce your risk of developing high blood pressure, type 2 diabetes, heart disease, and certain types of cancer. In a nutshell, physical activity improves the quality of your life and helps you live a longer, healthier life. I can't think of any better reasons to exercise than those.

What Kind of Exercise Is Best for Losing Weight?

When it comes to shedding weight, it is the total calories you burn during exercise that's most important. That's why cardiovascular exercises—the ones that get your heart beating faster for a continued period—are the best for promoting weight loss. Compared with strength and flexibility exercises, cardio or aerobic workouts burn more calories for the same duration of time. For example, for a person who weighs 150 pounds (68 kg), 30 minutes of yoga (which combines strength and flexibility exercises) burns roughly 180 calories, and a 30-minute moderate weight-training session burns about 235 calories. The same amount of cardiovascular exercise will burn more calories—238 if spinning, 275 if cross-country skiing, 306 if stair climbing, and 337 if jogging. The calorie burn from a cardio workout adds up over the course of the week, especially when it's combined with the No-Fail Diet.

To be most effective, cardio exercise needs to involve large muscle groups—your legs—and it needs to be maintained continuously. When you continuously exercise the big muscles in your legs, they use more oxygen than when they're not working. This challenges your cardiovascular system to deliver more oxygen to your working muscles. The end result? You burn extra calories and you get your heart, lungs, and circulatory system in shape. Here's a list of cardio exercises that will help you burn calories and lose weight:

Outside or at Home	At the Gym or Community Centre
aerobics video exercises	aerobics classes
brisk walking (3.8 to 4.2 miles/ 6.1 to 6.8 km per hour)	water aerobics classes
biking	brisk walking on a treadmill
cross-country skiing	circuit training
hiking	cross-country skiing on a ski machine
inline skating	cycling on a stationary bicycle
jogging	jogging on a treadmill
skipping rope	rowing on an ergometer
soccer	spinning classes
stair climbing	stair climbing on a StairMaster or stepmill
swimming laps	using an elliptical trainer
tennis, singles	

The total calories you burn during a cardio workout depends on the duration of the activity and the intensity (how hard you perform the exercise). If you walk briskly for 30 minutes, you'll burn about 200 calories. If you pick up your pace and jog instead, you'll burn an additional 140 calories. If you decide to tack on an extra 10 minutes to your usual half-hour jog, your muscles will use up 450 calories—an additional 110 calories.

The following table shows the estimated number of calories burned for various activities, performed at moderate (not vigorous) intensities, lasting 30 minutes. You'll notice that not all activities listed below are considered cardio workouts. I've included a variety of activities so you can see how they differ in terms of the energy your body uses to perform them. Calorie expenditures have been estimated for a 150 pound (68 kg) person. If you weigh more than that, you'll burn more calories, and if you're lighter, you'll burn less.

Calories Burned During 30 Minutes of Exercise

Activity	Calories Burned
Aerobics	202
Biking, on flat surface	220
Gardening	161
Golfing, no cart	130
Hiking	207

Housecleaning	121
Ice skating	207
Inline skating	238
Jogging	337
Kick-boxing	360
Mowing the lawn, hand pushed	162
Painting the house	171
Racquetball	220
Skiing, cross-country	274
Skiing, downhill	220
Spinning	238
Stair climbing	306
Swimming laps	301
Tennis, singles	274
Tennis, doubles	171
Walking briskly	198
Walking, with the dog	148
Water aerobics	144
Weight lifting	234
Yoga	180

Source: Calorie Control Council, www.caloriecontrol.org/exercalc.html.

The Benefits of Interval Training

A great way to increase your heart rate and burn more calories during cardiovascular exercise is to do interval training. Interval training constantly varies the intensity of exercise during your workout by alternating short, fast bursts of intensive exercise with slow, easy activity. For instance, you might walk briskly for 3 minutes, then run for 3 minutes, and keep alternating in this way for 20 to 30 minutes. If you work out on cardio machines, you can pick an interval-training program, or you can do it manually by increasing the resistance level or speed for short bursts. As you improve, you can slowly increase the intensity or duration, but not both at the same time.

Interval training helps improve your overall cardiovascular fitness by strengthening your heart and conditioning your muscles to better tolerate the buildup of lactic acid. (Lactic acid is a by-product of higher intensity exercise that causes a burning sensation in the muscles.) Interval training also helps prevent the injuries that often result from doing the same old repetitive cardiovascular exercise.

To help you get the best results from your exercise program—and to keep you interested—I've included a weekly interval workout in the No Fail 12-Week Fitness Program outlined in Chapter 5.

How Hard Should You Work Out?

Chances are you've heard the persistent myth that low-intensity aerobic workouts burn more body fat than do high-intensity workouts. It is true that at lower intensities of exercise your body's primary fuel source is fat, whereas at higher intensities you mainly burn glycogen, the sugars stored in your muscles and liver. But if you're burning fewer calories overall from a lower intensity workout, you won't lose weight as quickly. When it comes to losing body fat, the only thing that matters is how many calories you burn. Exercising at higher intensities will help you shed pounds faster because you burn more calories. You would have to exercise longer to get the same calorie burn from a low-intensity workout. In fact, some research suggests that exercising harder burns more calories both during and after your workout.

That's why those weight-loss or fat-loss programs on cardio machines at the gym are misleading. These preprogrammed workouts keep you exercising in a lower heart rate zone. That's fine if you have an hour to spend, but you'll get better results if you hit the cardio-fitness or interval-training programs that are designed to keep your heart beating faster.

Target Heart Rate Zone

To help you determine if you are working out in your target heart rate zone, you first need to figure out your maximum heart rate. Your maximum heart rate is the number of times your heart would beat in a minute if you were running as fast as you could. One way to estimate your maximum heart rate is to subtract your age from 220. However, this number can overestimate your maximum heart rate if you're under 40 and underestimate it if you're older. Researchers from the University of Colorado at Boulder recommend using this formula:

Maximum heart rate = 208 − (0.7 × your age)

So, if you're 40 years old, your maximum heart rate is 208 − (0.7 × 40) = 180 beats per minute.

If you're new to exercise, you should work out at between 50% to 70% of your maximum heart rate. To determine this range, multiply your maximum heart rate by 0.5 and by 0.7. A 40 year old with a maximum heart rate of 180 will have a target heart rate zone of 90 to 126 beats per minute (180 × 0.5 = 90 / 180 × 0.7 = 126).

If you already exercise regularly, aim for 70% to 90% of your maximum heart rate. A 40 year old with a maximum heart rate of 180 will need to be working out in a target heart rate zone of 126 to 162 beats per minute.

There are a few ways to figure out your heart rate during exercise. You can spend around $200 and buy a heart rate monitor, which consists of a band you wear around your chest that transmits your heart rate to a wristwatch. If you work out in a gym, you can also use the heart rate grips on cardio machines. They work best if your hands are slightly damp with sweat and your grip is light.

You can also do it the old-fashioned way by counting the number of times your heart beats in 10 seconds. Just hold two fingers (your pointer and middle fingers) to the inside of your wrist or on your neck. Once you find your pulse, look at the second hand of your watch and count the number of beats in 10 seconds (count from zero to 10). Now all you have to do is multiply that number by six to arrive at the beats per minute. If, during your workout, your heart beats 24 times in 10 seconds, that means it's beating 144 times per minute.

Rate of Perceived Exertion (RPE)

This is an alternate way to determine how hard you are working out, one that does not require counting your heart beats. This method relies on your perception of how hard you think you are exercising. You need to think about your breathing and muscle fatigue, or lack thereof. You must rate your overall discomfort on a scale from zero to 10. A rating of zero applies when you are at rest and not exerting yourself at all. A rating of 10 means you are exercising at an all-out-maximal effort and you can't work out any harder. Here are the definitions for each level of the RPE scale:

Level 0: This is the experience of total rest. You could sleep right now without a problem. Neither your heart rate nor your breathing is elevated. You will never be at this level during exercise.

Level 1: This is the feeling you would experience while watching TV. You are alert but there is no feeling of fatigue. Your thumb has the remote under complete control. It takes no effort on your behalf.

Level 2: This is the feeling you would experience while in the shower. You are awake and moving, but never briskly. You feel no fatigue or elevation in your heart rate or breathing.

Level 3: This is the feeling you would experience while moving about to do your day-to-day tasks. Your breathing feels natural and rhythmical.

Level 4: This is the feeling you would experience when you first start to warm up by walking slowly. Your breathing feels light.

Level 5: You are aware of your breathing. It is deeper than level 4 and you have slight fatigue.

Level 6: This is the feeling you would experience when you are behind in your schedule and running around. Your heart rate is elevated and you have a general feeling of fatigue, but you know you can maintain this level of exertion. (On the No-Fail 12-Week Fitness Program, this is what you want to experience at the end of your warm-up, during the active recovery phase of your Interval Cardio workout and during your Extended Cardio workout.)

Level 7: You are definitely breathing and there is definite fatigue. You are working hard at exercising vigorously. At this point you are pushing your limits. You could not keep this up all day but for the 15 minutes you have, you can push to it. It will be a challenge. (On the No-Fail 12-Week Fitness Program, this is the feeling you want to experience during your Standard Cardio workouts.)

Level 8: You have to tell yourself it is only for 2 minutes, then you can go back to an easier level. Working out at this level is a stretch for you to accomplish. When you are working at this level, ask yourself if you could do this for any longer than 2 minutes. If not, then you are at the right level. If you could, then you need to work a little harder. (This is the highest point you will be working toward. On the No-Fail 12-Week Fitness Program, you want to experience this level during the Work Phase of your Interval Cardio workouts.)

Level 9: Your breathing is very laboured and you could not maintain this level for more than a minute. You can't talk to your neighbour, not even one word.

Level 10: You should not experience level 10. You cannot maintain this for very long and there is no point in trying to.

In the cardio exercises in the No-Fail 12-Week Fitness Program in Chapter 5, you will be asked to start exercising at level 7 intensity for 15 minutes. (If this 15 minutes is too long for you exercise at this rate of perceived exertion, that's fine. Begin your workout at level 7 RPE and lower your intensity as you need to. Within a few weeks, as your fitness improves, you'll be able to exercise the entire time at level 7.) Remember, highly aerobic activity is not supposed to be comfortable. If you're able to read a magazine and talk on your cell phone while exercising, you're not working out hard enough. Challenge yourself.

Strength Training Counts Too

If you want to lose body fat, there's more to an exercise program than cardio alone. Sure it burns the most calories, but strength exercises that build muscular strength, tone, and endurance are also an important part of getting and staying lean. Strength training (also called resistance training) gives your muscles definition, reshapes problem areas, and increases your metabolism. It also improves your posture, prevents injuries, and can help reduce the risk of osteoporosis. The good news is that you don't need to spend hours at the gym lifting weights to see results. Research suggests that virtually all the health benefits of resistance training can be obtained in two 15-to-20-minute sessions per week.[2]

There are many ways to add resistance training to your fitness program:

At Home	At Home or the Gym	At the Gym or Community Centre
heavy yardwork	abdominal crunches	Cybex machines
raking and carrying leaves	chin-ups	free weights (dumbbells, barbells)
stair climbing	lunges	Nautilus machines
	push-ups	Pilates
	squats	spinning classes

What Are Reps and Sets?

Repetitions, or reps, refer to the number of times you do an exercise such as a leg lunge or bicep curl. A set is a group of repetitions. Depending on what your fitness goals are, you'll usually do one to three sets per strength exercise. You will improve your muscular fitness by performing only one set of a given exercise, but research suggests that optimal gains in strength and endurance are a result of multiple sets.

You need to break and rest your muscles for only 15 to 30 seconds between sets. Most of the recovery from muscle fatigue happens within the first 15 seconds. If you are new to exercise, take the full 30 seconds between sets; if you're experienced with weight training, take a 15-second rest only.

How Much Weight?

The amount of weight you lift will depend on your muscle strength and the number of reps you need to perform to achieve your goals.

Determining what weight to start at is a trial-and-error process. In general, you want to be able to feel the exercise by the time you are on the 8th or 9th repetition. The exercise should become difficult after 10 to 12 repetitions; you need to feel the resistance you are working against. The last 3 to 4 repetitions of the set should definitely challenge you. Your muscles should feel fatigued but you should not be in pain. You'll know the weight is right for you if it's a challenge to finish the exercise without compromising your form. If you have to contort your body in order to accomplish the last 3 or 4 repetitions, you need to reduce the amount of weight. You don't want the weight to be too heavy, but you also don't want it to be too light.

Flexibility for All-Round Fitness

Gentle reaching, bending, and stretching of your muscles help keep your joints flexible and your muscles relaxed. Being flexible means that your joints can move fluidly through a full range of motion. The more flexible you are, the less likely it is that you'll injure yourself during exercise. Being flexible helps reduce muscle soreness after exercise, improves posture, reduces back pain, and helps circulate nutrients and oxygen to muscles.

Unfortunately, stretching is often the most overlooked part of a fitness program. But the beauty of flexibility exercises is that they can be performed relatively quickly at any time of the day. It's easy to take a 5-minute stretch break in the middle of your day. You might not realize it, but many of the day-to-day activities you perform—vacuuming, yardwork, and gardening—help to maintain your flexibility, and certain sports—golf, bowling, and curling, for instance—have a flexibility component. Tai chi, yoga, and Pilates are fantastic ways to increase your flexibility.

The No-Fail 12-Week Fitness Program includes a series of simple stretching exercises that should be done after each cardiovascular workout. It's always best to stretch once your muscles are warmed up, as stretching with cold muscles may cause injury. Think of your muscles as being like plastic: difficult to stretch when cold, but add a little heat and the plastic becomes softer and more pliable. Your muscles behave the same way. During exercise, your muscles generate heat, becoming more pliable.

What's the Best Time to Exercise?

The answer to that question is any time of day that you can fit it in. The time of day you work out, whether in the morning, afternoon, or evening, has no bearing on how many calories you'll burn. That said, there are benefits to exercising first thing in the morning, before the day's distractions—a last-minute meeting, an inbox full of emails, or household chores—prevent you from sneaking in a workout. If you're a morning person, set your alarm earlier than usual so that you have time to exercise before leaving for work. If you have time to complete only part of your workout in the morning, you can finish the rest later in the day. If you're too busy getting kids ready for school to work out first thing, plan to exercise right after you drop them off at school. Many of my clients who are busy stay-at-home moms say they're much more likely to work out in the morning if they get dressed in their workout clothes. Once the kids head off to school, they're ready to power walk or head to the gym.

Studies do show that people who work out in the morning are far more likely to incorporate regular exercise into their lives over the long term. My clients tell me that a morning workout starts their day off on a positive note. They feel better about themselves and tend to make healthy food choices throughout the day. On the other hand, clients who wait until the end of a busy workday to exercise often lack the energy and motivation required to hit the gym.

Not everybody is a morning person, me included. I prefer to schedule my workouts for the mid- to late afternoon, when I am alert, energized, and in need of a distraction from my work. In fact, studies suggest that strength-training exercises are generally performed better when done in the afternoon or early evening. That's probably because during the course of the day our body temperature increases and our joints become looser.

What's most important is that you pick a time when your energy level is still high, when you feel motivated, and when you won't be distracted to do something else. If the only time you have to exercise is after dinner when the kids are asleep, so be it. That's likely going to be the time of day that you can stick with.

If You Truly Dislike Exercising

Let's face it: Some people just can't stand the thought of participating in any type of formal exercise. Perhaps you're one of them. Before you completely cross exercise off your to-do list, take a moment to reflect on the reasons why you dislike exercise. Make a list of all the obstacles preventing you from becoming physically active. You might be surprised to learn that there are ways to overcome perceived barriers. For instance, consider these obstacles, and their solutions:

• "Exercise is boring." You need to choose an activity that you think you will enjoy, one that feels more like play than exercise—for example, hiking, swimming, or a sports game, such as tennis or ultimate frisbee. To keep a fitness program interesting, you need to mix it up by adding a variety of activities to your routine. Combat boredom by trying different types of exercise classes or moving from the treadmill to the Stairmaster. If you fight with your brain to stay on the treadmill for 30 minutes, break up your routine: Jog for 15 minutes, then get on the stationary bike for the remaining 15 minutes. Perhaps you need to take a break from the gym and join a sports team. New exercises not only engage your mind, they also work different muscles and challenge your body. Last but not least, try listening to music or watching television while doing exercise.

• "I don't have time." While lack of time is a legitimate obstacle for many busy people, it's often used to explain away other barriers, such as not believing in your ability to exercise or feeling self-conscious in workout clothes. If you think that time really is the issue, take a few minutes to chart your downtime each day. How many hours do you spend watching television or surfing the internet? Logging your daily activities could illuminate possible time slots for exercise.

- "I don't like how I look right now." Concerns about appearance keep some people from exercising, especially those who think of themselves as sedentary. They feel self-conscious about their bodies and feel embarrassed in exercise clothes. "If I just lose a little weight first," they say, "I'll feel more comfortable going to the gym." Today, more and more facilities offer low-impact classes that cater to large-size people. Check out the exercise classes at your local community centre. If the thought of exercising with other people intimidates you, start exercising in the privacy of your home. Use exercise videos, a stationary bike, or a treadmill.

Exercise doesn't have to mean sweating buckets at the gym, on the tennis court, or on your treadmill at home. But you can, and should, become a little more active in your daily life. I call it the lifestyle approach to exercise. Your goal is to accumulate at least 30 minutes of moderate physical activity during the day. If you are not going for a run or taking an aerobics class, you must build activity into your daily routine. You won't lose weight as quickly, but short bouts of daily activity accumulate and can make a difference to your health and your waistline. Here are a few easy ways to accumulate 30 minutes' worth of lifestyle activity:

- Walk whenever you can—get off the bus a stop or two early, park at the far end of the lot, walk partway to work, or take the dog for an extra-long walk.

- Get a pedometer and use it. This device clips on to your belt or waistband and counts the number of steps you take each day. To be healthy, you need to take 10,000 steps per day; for weight loss you need to accumulate at least 12,000 steps.

- Use the stairs instead of the elevator, even if only for part of the way.

- Take the stairs instead of the escalator at the shopping mall.

- Avoid using walking sidewalks at airports.

- Ride your bicycle instead of driving to visit a neighbourhood friend.

- Walk at your lunch hour with co-workers or friends.
- Walk to visit a co-worker instead of sending an email.
- Play actively with your kids.
- Get up off the couch and stretch for a few minutes each hour.
- Ride a stationary bicycle while watching TV.
- On the golf course, carry or push your golf bag instead of riding in a cart.

Staying Motivated

The decision to get and stay physically fit requires a lifelong commitment of both time and effort. Exercising and eating healthfully must become things you do naturally every day, like brushing your teeth. And you need to be patient. Don't try to do too much too soon or you'll give up before you get a chance to reap the rewards. Some days will be harder than others. It's on those days that you need to focus on your goals and remind yourself why you're doing this.

Add Variety

If you perceive your workout as a chore, you more than likely won't stick with it. Keep it interesting by planning different types of cardio workouts each week—a power walk with a friend, a fitness class at the gym, and a hike on the weekend. There is no rule that says you have to get on that treadmill 4 days a week to stay fit. If you find your weight-training program is getting boring, mix things up. Vary how often you do an exercise and the number of sets and reps you do. Find an alternate exercise that works the same muscles. Instead of doing your bicep curls with dumbbells, try doing them on a weight machine at the gym. Instead of doing two sets of bicep curls back to back, do one and then immediately do one set of tricep exercises, followed by one set of shoulders exercises. When you're done, repeat the circuit to complete your second set of each exercise.

Schedule Your Workouts

Record your workout schedule in your BlackBerry, Palm Pilot, day planner, or kitchen calendar. Schedule your exercise times just like you would any other appointment, and stick to these times. Remember, you are just as important as any other person that you schedule in during your day. If you can, schedule exercise on the same days and at the same time so that workouts become a natural part of your life, not something that happens only if you get around to it.

Find a Workout Partner

Many people find they are more likely to exercise if they have a friend to exercise with. If you're having trouble motivating yourself to get out the door, ask a friend or family member to join you. Even if you don't feel like exercising, having someone to walk, jog, or bike with will increase your motivation and make the time go by faster. Or try a group exercise class. Working out with people who share a common goal can be a big motivator.

Keep a Fitness Journal

In Appendix 1, page 343, you'll find a 12-Week Fitness Tracker. Use this to record your daily activity and workouts each week. You'll be surprised how motivating it is to watch your fitness improve over time. Use your journal to reflect on what activities you've done for the past few weeks. Doing so provides a sense of accomplishment and encourages you to keep going.

Hire a Certified Personal Trainer

Working with a personal trainer motivates me to do my weight workouts. For starters, I have someone waiting for me, so I have to show up even if I don't feel like it. But a trainer also makes me work harder than I would on my own, and seeing my progress inspires me to keep on exercising. I also enjoy the company as I work out.

You might want to hire a personal trainer only once or twice to show you the ropes and get you started. Or you might prefer weekly sessions to keep you focused. If you belong to a health club, there are bound to be a few personal trainers on staff. If you work out at home and would like the help of a personal trainer, the Certified Professional Trainers Network can refer you to a professional in your community. Visit its website at www.cptn.com.

3

Foods for Health and Longevity

Losing weight is not just about fitting into a smaller pair of jeans. It's true that looking and feeling good in your clothes will give you a big boost in self-confidence. And that's important. But losing weight is also about improving your health. In fact, personal health is the number one reason why many of my clients decide to start a weight-loss program. Some people want to shed excess pounds to improve their blood test results—they're motivated to lower their cholesterol or blood sugar levels. Others see losing weight as a way to reduce their blood pressure and, hopefully, discontinue their blood pressure pills. Some of my clients are tired of living with constant knee and back pain and understand that a lighter body weight will ease much of their discomfort. Still others who suffer from obstructive sleep apnea are encouraged to lose weight to improve their sleep. (Sleep apnea is a disorder in which complete or partial obstruction of the airway during sleep causes loud snoring, disrupted sleep, and excessive daytime sleepiness.)

There's no question that losing excess body fat can improve your health in many ways. Even if you don't have high cholesterol, hypertension, or sleep apnea, achieving a healthy weight can reduce your risk of developing certain health problems, including heart disease, type 2 diabetes, and some cancers. But there's more to improving your health than just slimming down, and it has to do with what you put in your mouth. It's possible to reach your healthy weight goal by following any number of diets. But depending on what foods those diets encourage you to eat, or to avoid, you might be jeopardizing your health and your nutrient intake.

Not long ago Jill, a 38-year-old stay-at-home mom, came to see me for help lowering her blood cholesterol. Jill had always received a clean bill of health from her doctor after every checkup—except for this year when she was told her blood cholesterol had jumped to a very high number. Jill's doctor promptly referred her to me for nutrition counselling. Once I analyzed Jill's diet it became pretty obvious what was contributing to her elevated cholesterol reading: She ate too many foods packed with saturated (animal) fat. Jill added 18% cream to her numerous cups of coffee, she snacked on cheese, she ate salami (and more cheese) sandwiches for lunch, and she added butter to bread and vegetables.

She told me these fatty foods were remnants of a high-protein, low-carb diet she had followed the previous year—a diet that helped her lose 10 pounds but encouraged her to eat high-fat animal foods. Eventually the carbs crept back in, but, unfortunately, the high-fat foods remained. One year after following this high-protein diet, Jill sat in my office with a cholesterol problem and her 10 pounds back on. I revamped her diet, and she was able to lower her cholesterol level and take off those unwanted pounds.

If you're going to lose weight, it's important to do it properly. That means eating those foods that will help you achieve your weight goal and improve your health, possibly even increase your longevity. The No-Fail Diet is a weight-loss plan that teaches you how to eat right for long-term health. It's a meal plan that includes foods that are scientifically proven to help reduce the risk of developing high blood pressure, heart disease, stroke, type 2 diabetes, and certain cancers. Combined with the 12-Week No-Fail Fitness Program, you'll be well on the way to a slimmer, healthier you.

In Chapter 4, you'll learn all about the No-Fail Diet food groups and the healthiest food choices within each. On the No-Fail Diet you will make smart food choices—choosing foods that are low in saturated and trans fats, low in refined sugars, high in fibre and whole grains, and packed with vitamins, minerals, and disease-fighting plant chemicals. Now it's time to explain the 10 nutrition tenets that will guide your food choices on the No-Fail Diet—as well as the food choices you make over the long term.

Choose Foods Low in Saturated Fat

Over the past two decades, high-fat diets have been blamed for obesity, heart disease, and cancer. Until recently, health agencies advocated the 30% rule: Limit fat intake to no more than 30% of your daily calories. We were told to eat less fat to help us lose weight, lower our cholesterol levels, and possibly even ward off cancer. But this simple recommendation to follow a low-fat diet is now largely out of date. Recent studies suggest that certain fats can help lower blood pressure, fatty nuts reduce the risk of type 2 diabetes, and oil-based salad dressings guard against heart disease. Today, a healthy diet can actually contain as much as 35% of its calories from fat—provided, of course, you choose the right fats. What matters most when it comes to your health is the *type* of fat you eat. All fats are not created equal: Some fats increase the risk of health problems, whereas other fats can decrease the risk.

When it comes to weight loss, however, *all* fats are equal—identical in calories, that is. One gram of fat—be it fat from butter, olive oil, or margarine—contains 9 calories. That means that 1 tablespoon (15 ml) of butter or vegetable oil provides roughly 120 calories. As far as your waistline is concerned, it makes no difference where those fat calories come from—they're all treated the same. And since 1 gram of fat delivers more than double the calories found in the same portion of carbohydrate or protein, fat calories can add up fast if you're not careful. The bottom line: Choosing foods that are lower in fat *and* limiting the quantity of fats and oils you add to your foods can help reduce the number of calories you eat, and ultimately will help you lose weight.

For this reason, you won't be eating heaps of salad dressing, butter, or olive oil on the No-Fail Diet, but you will be allowed a little each day. As well, your food choices will focus on limiting the so-called bad fats while emphasizing the good fats. Here's how the type of fat you eat can impact your health:

Saturated versus Unsaturated Fats

Fats are classified as saturated, monounsaturated, or polyunsaturated, based on which type of fat is present in the greatest concentration. (Dietary fats are really a mixture of saturated, polyunsaturated, and monounsaturated fatty acids, but we call them by the name of the fatty acid they have the most of.) *Saturated fat* is found in animal foods including beef, veal, lamb, pork, lard, poultry fat, butter, cream, whole milk, and cheese. Plant oils such as coconut, palm kernel oil, and palm oil are also highly saturated. Saturated fats contribute to the risk of heart disease by raising LDL, or bad, cholesterol. Some studies have also linked a diet high in saturated fat with an increased risk of prostate cancer.

Vegetable oils, nuts, and seeds are the main dietary source of *unsaturated* fats, also known as *polyunsaturated* and *monounsaturated* fats. Safflower oil, sunflower oil, corn oil, walnuts, Brazil nuts, and seeds contain high levels of polyunsaturated fats. Olive oil, canola oil, peanut oil, avocado, almonds, and hazelnuts contain more monounsaturated fats. Both polyunsaturated and monounsaturated fats help lower blood cholesterol when they're used in place of cholesterol-raising saturated fats. Olive oil's heart-healthy reputation might also be due to a naturally occurring anti-inflammatory chemical called oleocanthal.

Omega-3 Fats

These fats belong to the family of polyunsaturated fats. Cold water fish such as salmon, lake trout, sardines, mackerel, and herring contain two omega-3 fats: DHA (docosahexaenoic acid) and EPA (eicosapentaenoic acid). No doubt you've heard that eating oily fish a few times each week can help reduce your risk of heart attack and stroke. That's because omega-3 fats help make blood less likely to form clots and protect against irregular heartbeats that cause sudden cardiac death. Omega-3 fats may do more than keep our hearts healthy. Research suggests that fish oils can block the growth of certain types of tumours and may slow the onset of age-related dementia. (Omega-3 fatty acids, especially DHA, help keep the lining of brain cells flexible so memory messages can pass easily between cells. Our brain cells continuously need to refresh themselves with a new supply of omega-3 fats.)

Flaxseed, walnut, and canola oils contain another omega-3 fat, ALA (alpha-linolenic acid). ALA is called an essential fatty acid because our bodies can't make it on their own and so it must be obtained from our diet. Consuming oils rich in ALA may be good for the heart, particularly in women. A recent study found that, among 76,763 healthy women who were followed for 18 years, those who consumed the most ALA had a 40% lower risk of sudden cardiac death compared with women whose diets provided the least.[1]

Being Fat Smart on the No-Fail Diet

As you work toward your weight goal, you will choose foods that are low in saturated fat. And the fats that you add to your foods— vegetable oils, salad dressings, and spreads—will be primarily composed of heart-healthy poly- and monounsaturated fats. On the No-Fail Diet you will also be encouraged to eat fish at least twice weekly. (That's why I have included two fish meals per week in the No-Fail Diet Menu Plans in Chapter 6.)

Choose Animal Foods That Are Low in Saturated Fat

The following is a list of animal foods that are lower in saturated fat and which are included in the No-Fail Diet's food groups:

Total Fat and Saturated Fat of Selected Foods (Grams)

Total Fat		Saturated Fat
Dairy Products		
Cheddar cheese, low-fat, 7% MF,* 1 oz (30 g)	2.0	1.2
Cottage cheese, 1% MF, 1/2 cup (125 ml)	1.1	0.8
Cottage cheese, fat-free, 1/2 cup (125 ml)	0.5	0.3
Mozzarella cheese, part-skim, 16.5% MF, 1 oz (30 g)	4.6	2.9
Milk, 1% MF, 1 cup (250 ml)	2.5	1.7
Milk, skim, 0.1% MF, 1 cup (250 ml)	0.5	0.3
Frozen yogurt, vanilla, 5.6% MF, 1/2 cup (125 ml)	4.0	2.5

Meat and Poultry

Beef, steak, eye of round, grilled, 3 oz (90 g)	7.7	2.7
Beef, steak, inside round, grilled, 3 oz (90 g)	3.9	1.4
Beef, steak, top sirloin, grilled, 3 oz (90 g)	6.8	2.6
Beef, tenderloin, roasted, 3 oz (90 g)	7.3	2.3
Ground beef patty, extra-lean, broiled, 3 oz (90 g)	7.8	2.1
Pork, back (peameal) bacon, grilled, 3 oz (90 g)	7.5	2.5
Pork, ham, lean, 5% fat, 3 oz (90 g)	4.8	1.6
Pork tenderloin, roasted, 3 oz (90 g)	3.2	1.0
Veal, ground, broiled, 3 oz (90 g)	6.8	2.7
Veal, grain-fed, lean loin chop, broiled, 3 oz (90 g)	5.7	2.4
Veal, sirloin, roasted, 3 oz (90 g)	5.6	2.2
Veal, grain-fed, cutlets, pan fried, 3 oz (90 g)	2.5	0.8
Chicken breast, roasted, skinless, 3 oz (90 g)	1.9	0.6
Chicken, dark meat, roasted, skinless, 3 oz (90 g)	8.7	2.4
Chicken, white meat, roasted, skinless, 3 oz (90 g)	4.0	1.1
Turkey, dark meat, roasted, skinless, 3 oz (90 g)	2.7	0.9
Turkey, white meat, roasted, skinless, 3 oz (90 g)	0.9	0.2
Eggs		
Egg whites, 2 large	0	0
Egg, whole, 1 large	5.3	1.6

* milk fat

Source: Health Canada, Canadian Nutrient File, 2005; www.healthcanada.ca/cnf

Choose Poly- and Monounsaturated Fats in Food Preparation

When using added fats and oils in food preparation, choose poly- and monounsaturated fats. Try to avoid saturated fats.

Polyunsaturated Fats	Monounsaturated Fats	Saturated Fats
corn oil	avocado	butter
safflower oil	canola oil	cheese spreads
sesame oil	olive oil	cream cheese
soybean oil	olives	lard
sunflower oil	peanut oil	solid shortening
walnut oil	almonds	macadamia nuts

Polyunsaturated Fats	Monounsaturated Fats
margarines made from these oils	cashews
Brazil nuts	filberts
pumpkin seeds	peanuts
sesame seeds	pecans
sunflower seeds	pistachios
walnuts	

Find Fat on Nutrition Labels

Start reading the Nutrition Facts box on prepackaged foods. This will help you in shopping for lower fat foods. Look at the grams of total fat per serving stated on the label. This information is listed after the calories per serving.

```
Nutrition Facts
Per 1 cup (264g)
─────────────────────────────
Amount                % Daily Value
─────────────────────────────
Calories 260
─────────────────────────────
Fat 13g                      20%
─────────────────────────────
  Saturated Fat 3g
  + Trans Fat 2g             25%
─────────────────────────────
Cholesterol 30mg
─────────────────────────────
Sodium 660mg                 28%
─────────────────────────────
Carbohydrate 31g             10%
─────────────────────────────
  Fibre 0g                    0%
─────────────────────────────
  Sugars 5g
─────────────────────────────
Protein 5g
─────────────────────────────
Vitamin A 4%  •  Vitamin C 2%
Calcium 15%  •  Iron 4%
```

For example, the nutrition label shown above tells you that a 1 cup (264 g) serving of this particular food provides 13 grams of fat. Use this information to help you choose between different brands of crackers, cookies, cereals, frozen dinners, soups, and snack foods: It's an easy way to select lower fat brands. Where possible, choose a product that provides no more than 3 grams of fat for every 100 calories (this means the product has no more than 30% fat calories).

You'll notice that fat, and saturated fat plus trans fat, are also expressed as a percentage of daily value (% DV). (You'll learn more about trans fat, another bad fat, in the next section.) Daily values are based on recommended intakes. The % DV helps you quickly evaluate whether there's a little or a lot of a particular nutrient in 1 serving of the food. In the case of fat, the daily value is set at 65 grams, which includes 20 grams of saturated fat plus trans fat. Look for products that have a % DV of 10% or less for saturated plus trans fats; that means they will be low in these bad fats. Foods with a % DV of 25% or more for saturated plus trans fats are very high in these fats—avoid buying them.

Choose Foods That Contain Little or No Trans Fat

Trans fats are formed when vegetable oils are processed into margarine or shortening. This chemical process, called partial hydrogenation, adds hydrogen atoms to liquid vegetable oils, making them more solid and therefore more useful to food manufacturers. Cookies, crackers, pastries, and muffins made with partially hydrogenated vegetable oils are more palatable and have a longer shelf life. A margarine that's made by hydrogenating a vegetable oil is firmer, like butter.

Partial hydrogenation makes a fat become saturated, and it forms a new type of fat called *trans fat*. Hydrogenation also destroys essential fatty acids that your body needs from unprocessed vegetable oils. Like saturated fat found in meat and dairy, a steady intake of trans fat can increase your total and LDL cholesterol numbers. But unlike saturated fat, consuming too much trans fat can lower your HDL (good) cholesterol. Compared with saturated fats, trans fats are linked with a 2.5- to 10-fold higher risk of heart disease. The harmful effects of trans fats aren't limited to heart disease. Research also suggests that diets high in trans fat increase the risk of type 2 diabetes.

Over the past 50 years, industry-produced trans fat has become a common ingredient in hundreds of popular foods. You'll find trans fat in foods that list partially hydrogenated vegetable oil and/or shortening as ingredients. Roughly 90% of the trans fat in our food supply lurks in commercial baked goods, snack foods, fried fast foods, and some margarines. Trans fat occurs naturally in beef and dairy products, but in tiny amounts. It's also not known if trans fat in beef and dairy behaves the same way in the body as industry-produced trans fat.

Foods that are made with *fully* hydrogenated vegetable oils are high in saturated fat, but they do not contain trans fats. Unfortunately, both partially hydrogenated oils and fully hydrogenated oils are often listed the same way on labels—as hydrogenated oils. Because of this, the only way to tell if trans fat is present in a food is to read the Nutrition Facts table. When buying packaged foods, choose products that contain less than 0.5 grams of trans fat per serving, and ideally none.

In September 2002, the National Academy of Sciences (a panel of Canadian and American experts) issued a report stating there is no safe level of trans fat. While it is impossible to avoid all trans fat, your intake should be as low as possible. The foods you will eat on the No-Fail Diet do not contain any foods made with partially hydrogenated vegetable oil or shortening. In the No-Fail Diet Menu Plan, I occasionally recommend brand name products, to help you save time in the kitchen. But rest assured, these products are trans fat free. (To be labelled "free of trans fat," a product must contain less than 0.2 grams of trans fat per serving *and* it must have no more than 2 grams of trans and saturated fat combined.)

Choose Whole-Grain Foods More Often

There are plenty of reasons to trade in your white bread for whole-wheat, your white rice for brown, and your Rice Krispies for Cheerios. Studies have found that whole-grain eaters have a lower risk of heart disease, type 2 diabetes, obesity, and certain cancers than do their peers who fill up on refined grains. A steady intake of whole grains may even slow the progression of heart disease. One study from Tufts University in Boston found that among postmenopausal women with established heart disease, those who consumed more than 6 servings of whole grains per week had decreased narrowing of the coronary arteries compared with women who consumed fewer whole grains.[2]

Whole-grain foods are made from the entire grain seed—the outer bran layer where nearly all the fibre is; the germ layer, rich in vitamins and minerals; and the endosperm, which contains the starch. Whole grains can be eaten whole, cracked, split, flaked, or ground. Often they're milled into flour and used to make breads, cereals, pastas, and crackers. A whole grain can be a single food, such as oatmeal, brown rice, flaxseed, popcorn, kamut, millet, or quinoa, or it can be an ingredient in another food such as bread, crackers, or breakfast cereal.

The health benefits of whole grains go beyond fibre. Whole grains contain a package of nutrients that includes vitamins, minerals, fibre, and hundreds of phytochemicals, natural compounds that have health benefits. The individual components of whole grains are thought to work together to guard against disease.

When whole grains are refined, most of the bran and germ is stripped away. As a result, refined grains contain significantly less fibre, B vitamins, vitamin E, calcium, magnesium, and potassium, and 75% fewer phytochemicals than their unrefined counterparts. Refined grains are enriched with some, but not all, vitamins and minerals lost through processing. But disease-fighting phytochemicals are not added back.

Knowing what's a whole grain and what's not can be challenging, and you won't always find this information on nutrition labels of food packages. To help, here's a list of selected grains and grain products:

Whole Grains	Refined Grains
brown rice	cornmeal
bulgur	pasta, white
corn	pearl barley
emmer	rice flour
farro	rye flour
flaxseed	wheat flour
kamut	wheat flour, unbleached
kasha (buckwheat groats)	white rice
millet	
oat bran	
oatmeal	
popcorn	

Whole Grains

pot barley
quinoa
spelt
wheat berries
whole and cracked wheat
whole rye
wild rice

There's no official recommended intake for whole grains, but I recommend that you eat at least 3 servings per day. This is the amount that's linked with protection from many diseases and may even help you control your weight (whole grains keep you feeling full longer than refined grains so you end up eating less). The following tips will help you increase your intake of whole grains (you'll also find many whole-grain foods and recipes on the No-Fail Diet Menu Plan):

- Read food packaging labels carefully. Look for claims such as "100% whole grain whole wheat" or "made with 100% whole grains." Foods that simply state "whole grains" may contain only small amounts.

- Read the ingredient list on breads, crackers, and breakfast cereals. Look for a whole grain to be listed first. This means that the product is predominately whole grain. If a whole grain is listed second, you might be getting only a little or only half whole grain. If you checked the ingredient list on your box of 100% bran cereal, you might be surprised to learn that it is not made from whole grains. However, you can consider these cereals as whole grain since they are a concentrated source of bran that's missing from refined grains.

- Try pasta made from whole wheat, spelt, or kamut.

- Substitute bulgur, quinoa, or wild or brown rice for potatoes and white rice.

- Sneak whole grains into recipes—add oatmeal to pancakes, flaxseed to muffins, bulgur and barley to soups and stews.

- Replace half the white flour with whole-wheat flour in recipes for baked goods.

Choose Low Glycemic Carbohydrate Foods More Often

Many popular diets are based on the concept of the glycemic index (GI). The GI is a relatively new concept in the world of carbohydrates. It's a scale that ranks carbohydrate-rich foods by how fast they raise blood sugar levels compared with pure glucose (the simplest form of sugar), which is ranked 100. The lower a food's glycemic index value, the less potent are its effects on your blood sugar.

Foods with a high GI value are digested quickly and cause a rapid rise in blood sugar, and therefore, an outpouring of insulin (the hormone that removes sugar from your blood and stores it in cells). This surge of insulin can trigger hunger and overeating. A steady intake of fast-acting carbohydrates can lead to chronic high insulin levels and eventually insulin resistance, a precursor for type 2 diabetes.

Foods that are ranked high on the GI scale (70 or higher) include white bread, whole-wheat bread, baked russet potatoes, refined breakfast cereals, instant oatmeal, cereal bars, Pop-Tarts, raisins, dates, ripe bananas, carrots, honey, and white sugar.

Foods with a low GI value (less than 55) release their sugar more slowly into the bloodstream and don't produce a rush of insulin. Examples of low GI foods are grainy breads with seeds, steel-cut and long-cooking oats, 100% bran cereals, brown rice, sweet potatoes, pasta, apples, citrus fruit, grapes, pears, legumes, nuts, seeds, milk, yogurt, and soy milk.

Studies suggest that diets based on low glycemic carbohydrates can help prevent type 2 diabetes and colon cancer. Experiments have even shown that eating a meal comprising low GI carbohydrates can prevent overeating later in the day. The prolonged presence of slowly digested carbohydrates in your stomach can stimulate receptors that tell your brain you're full. You stop eating sooner and feel satisfied longer. That said, there is no evidence to show that a low glycemic diet promotes weight loss.

Nevertheless, most foods with a low glycemic index are very nutritious. Many are high in fibre and most are packed with vitamins and minerals. And the fact that low GI foods are linked with protection from type 2 diabetes and colon cancer makes them very worthwhile foods to add to your diet. That's why they are included in the No-Fail Diet. Aim to include at least one low GI food per meal, or base two of your meals on low GI choices. But there's no need to carry around a calculator or memorize a lengthy list of GI food values. Here are a few much simpler ways to ensure you're eating a diet that consists mainly of low GI foods:

- Use common sense. Unprocessed fresh foods—whole grains, legumes, nuts, fruits, and vegetables—have a low GI value. High glycemic foods are usually highly processed and may have a concentrated amount of refined sugar.

- Pay attention to breads and breakfast cereals, since these foods contribute the most to the high glycemic value of our North American diet.

- Avoid eating high GI snacks such as pretzels, corn chips, and rice cakes, as these can trigger hunger and overeating. Snacks on the No-Fail Diet include fresh fruit, low-fat dairy products, soy milk, nuts, and plain popcorn.

- Include fruits that are more acidic (oranges, grapefruit, cherries) in your daily diet, as these have a low GI and will lower the total GI of a meal.

- Use salad dressings made from vinegar or lemon juice—the acidity will result in a further reduction in the total GI of your meal.

There's another reason why I don't think it's necessary to base your food choices solely on a list of GI values. I've met many clients who have taken the concept of glycemic index to the extreme, avoiding healthy and nutrient-packed foods just because their GI numbers are high. If you limit your diet to include only foods with a low GI value, you'll miss out on important nutrients found in some higher GI foods. Take whole-wheat bread, for example. It's definitely a more nutritious choice than fluffy white bread, but because both are finely milled, they both have a high GI. Carrots also have a high GI but are loaded with cancer-fighting beta-carotene. The same goes for bananas and dates, two fruits that are high on the GI scale. Bananas are loaded with potassium, and dates are an excellent source of magnesium, two minerals linked with healthy blood pressure. On the flipside, not all low GI foods are good for you. Ice cream has a GI value of 38 but it's packed with saturated fat. White chocolate scores a 44, but it's loaded with sugar.

The bottom line: Keep the glycemic index in perspective. GI values are based on eating a single food on an empty stomach. Meal size, fat content of your meal, and the variety of foods eaten together will skew the glycemic index.

Limit Your Refined Sugar Intake

If you read food labels, you've seen them listed as dextrose, liquid sugar, honey, fructose, molasses, and by a handful of other names. More and more, added sugars are finding their way into the foods we eat. And it's not just the usual suspects such as soft drinks, candy, cookies, and cakes that contain sugars. Sugars lurk in salad dressings, frozen dinners, pasta sauces, soy milk, peanut butter, and bread.

Even if you don't have a sweet tooth, you might be consuming more sugar than you think—and more than is good for you. There's no evidence that sugar causes diabetes, heart disease, cancer, or hyperactivity, but too much can wreak havoc on your health in other ways. A steady intake of sugar adds a surplus of calories to your diet, extra calories that can lead to weight gain if you don't burn them off.

Added sugars, as the name implies, are those added to foods during processing and preparation. They're disguised under many names on ingredient lists: brown sugar, corn syrup, dextrose, fructose, high-fructose corn syrup, fruit juice concentrate, glucose-fructose, honey, invert sugar, liquid sugar, malt, maltose, molasses, rice syrup, table sugar, and sucrose. Manufacturers add sugars to foods for reasons that go beyond making them taste sweet. Sugars act as a preservative, enhance flavour, add bulk and texture, and aid in the browning of foods. Added sugars are not to be confused with naturally occurring sugars, such as lactose in milk and yogurt and fructose in fruit and sweet vegetables.

The most controversial added sugar is high-fructose corn syrup, a sweetener that's added to soft drinks, fruit drinks, baked goods, and canned fruit. Researchers have linked our increased use of corn syrup sweeteners over the past 20 years with rising obesity rates. This correlation certainly doesn't prove that high-fructose corn syrup causes weight gain. But some experts contend that fructose in high-fructose corn syrup is processed differently by our bodies than is glucose in cane or beet sugar. Fructose doesn't trigger hormone responses that regulate appetite and satiety, which could trick you into overeating.

How can you tell if you're eating too much added sugar? A spoonful of sugar is easy to spot but other sugars are not, especially those hidden away in everyday foods. You need to read labels to sleuth out hidden sugars. The Nutrition Facts box on prepackaged foods discloses the grams of sugars contained in 1 serving of the food. You can do the math to convert grams of sugars to teaspoons of sugar: 1 teaspoon (5 ml) of sugar has 4 grams of sugar. But keep in mind that the sugar numbers on nutrition labels include both naturally occurring sugars (e.g., fruit or milk sugars) and refined sugars added during food processing (e.g., sucrose, honey, corn syrup).

Cutting back on added sugars is one strategy that can help you lose weight. The following tips will help you curb your intake of— and burn off—added sugars. (You won't find any foods high in added sugars in the No-Fail Diet.)

- Limit sugary drinks. Replace soft drinks and fruit drinks (e.g., fruit punch, Fruitopia, Five Alive) with water, low-fat milk, vegetable juice, or tea.

- Satisfy your sweet tooth with natural sugars. Choose fruit, yogurt, or smoothies over candy, cakes, cookies, and pastries.

- Think small. Avoid the temptation to order king-size desserts, pastries, and candy bars when eating away from home. Although you will be allowed to indulge in a weekly treat while following the No-Fail Diet, I recommend that you stick with a moderate portion size.

- Choose breakfast cereals that have no more than 8 grams of sugar per serving. Exceptions include cereals with dried fruit and 100% bran cereals.

- Sweeten foods with spices instead of sugar. Add cinnamon and nutmeg to hot cereals, a dash of vanilla to coffee and lattes, and grated fresh ginger to cut fruit and vegetables.

- Reduce sugar in recipes. As a general rule, you can cut the sugar in most baked goods recipes by one-third.

- Get moving. Aim to get 30 minutes of physical activity every day. The No-Fail 12-Week Fitness Program, discussed in Chapter 5, will help you do just that.

Eat Plenty of Fruits and Vegetables Each Day

No doubt you've been told since childhood to eat your fruits and vegetables—and for good reason. Nutritionists like me have long praised the health benefits of a diet packed with produce. Over the past few decades, hundreds and hundreds of studies have linked a high intake of fruits and vegetables to protection from cancers, heart attack, stroke, and high blood pressure. Research even suggests that boosting your intake of fruits and vegetables may help preserve your eyesight as you age.

We don't yet know all the reasons why fruits and vegetables help keep us healthy, but researchers have pinned down a number of their protective compounds, including the nutrients folate, vitamins C and A, calcium, and magnesium, as well as dietary fibre. Produce also contains literally hundreds of phytochemicals, natural compounds such as beta-carotene, lutein, lycopene, and flavonoids, which act as antioxidants and protect our cells from the harmful effects of free radicals.

Despite the overwhelming evidence that fruits and vegetables are good for us, many of us still fall short of the recommended 7 to 10 servings per day. It's estimated that only 30% of Canadians eat at least 5 daily servings. Seven to 10 servings might sound like a lot, but a serving size isn't that large. If it fits in your hand, it's probably 1 serving—a medium-size fruit, 1/4 cup (50 ml) dried fruit, 1/2 cup (125 ml) cooked vegetables, 1 cup (250 ml) salad, or 1/2 cup (125 ml) vegetable or fruit juice.

If you forgo your fruits and vegetables until the end of the day, you won't come close to meeting your target. The key is to incorporate fruits and vegetables into all of your meals and snacks. Here's how you'll increase your intake on the No-Fail Diet:

- *At breakfast include 1 fruit serving.* Toss chopped banana, raisins, or dried cranberries into a bowl of whole-grain cereal. Or purée frozen blueberries and strawberries with low-fat milk or soy milk to make a breakfast fruit smoothie. Or enjoy a small glass of unsweetened citrus juice with your morning meal. The vitamin C enhances iron absorption from the whole grains.

- *Add vegetables to your lunch.* Add sliced tomatoes, cucumbers, grated carrot, and lettuce to your sandwich. Try spinach leaves as a change from lettuce. Add a handful of baby carrots or strips of bell peppers to your brown-bag lunch. If you buy your lunch from the deli, order a small vegetable soup with your sandwich. Replace diet pop with lycopene-packed tomato or vegetable juice.

- *Carry fruit with you for a midday snack.* Keep a bowl of fresh fruit on your kitchen counter and in your office. If you're bored of apples and bananas, pack a single-serving can of unsweetened fruit or applesauce in your briefcase. Or prepare snack-size bags of dried apricots, raisins, and almonds. Midday snacks can also include carrot sticks, cherry tomatoes, red bell pepper strips, broccoli florets, and mushroom caps with hummus or a low-fat creamy dip.

- *Include at least 2 vegetable servings at dinner.* Use romaine and other dark green lettuces in salads (they've got more beta-carotene than iceberg lettuce). Bake, microwave, or boil a sweet potato for a change from the usual white potato or white rice. Add quick-cooking greens such as spinach, kale, rapini, or Swiss chard to soups and pasta sauces. Roast or grill eggplant, peppers, asparagus, fennel, onion, and mushrooms. Add the leftovers to tomorrow's lunch.

- *Choose fruits and vegetables based on colour.* To consume a wide variety of nutrients and protective plant compounds, include at least two different coloured fruits and three different coloured vegetables each day. Think dark green and orange.

- *Take advantage of convenient pre-prepped produce* sold in the grocery store if you're short on time. You'll find fresh fruit salad, peeled and cored fresh pineapple, and individual serving sizes of raisins, dried fruit bars, and canned fruit (buy fruit canned in its own juice or water, rather than in syrup). You'll find ready-to-eat salads, carrot sticks, broccoli florets, stir-fry vegetables, shredded cabbage, grated carrot, triple-washed fresh spinach, and cubed turnip and squash.

- *Don't discount frozen vegetables,* especially when you're buying produce that's out of season. Considering that some produce arrives at the grocery store up to 2 weeks after harvest and often sits on the shelf (or in your refrigerator) for some time thereafter, frozen produce can actually be higher in nutrients than fresh because it's flash-frozen immediately after picking. (When fresh fruits and vegetables are exposed to light and air, the vitamins in them break down over time.)

Leslie's Top Picks in the Produce Department

Good source of ...	Top produce picks ...
Folate, a B vitamin that may help protect from heart disease and certain cancers	Artichokes, asparagus, avocado, beets, Brussels sprouts, romaine lettuce, spinach
Vitamin C, an antioxidant that may help ward off cataracts	Cantaloupe, grapefruit, kiwi, mangoes, oranges, strawberries, tomato juice, bell peppers, broccoli, Brussels sprouts, cauliflower
Beta-carotene, an antioxidant linked with protection from lung cancer, cataracts, and macular degeneration	Apricots, cantaloupe, mangoes, nectarines, peaches, broccoli, carrots, collard greens, kale, pumpkin, spinach, sweet potato, winter squash
Anthocyanins, phytochemicals being studied for their anti-aging properties	Blackberries, blueberries, blackcurrants, plums, purple grapes, raisins, eggplant, purple cabbage, purple carrots, purple peppers
Cruciferous compounds, phytochemicals that help the body detoxify carcinogens	Bok choy, broccoli, Brussels sprouts, cabbage, cauliflower, collard greens, kale, rutabaga, turnip

Lutein, a phytochemical that may reduce the risk of cataract and macular degeneration	Grapes, kiwi, beet greens, broccoli, collard greens, kale, okra, red bell peppers, spinach, Swiss chard, zucchini
Lycopene, a phytochemical linked with protection from prostate cancer	Canned tomatoes, tomato juice, tomato paste, guava, pink grapefruit, watermelon

Reduce Your Daily Sodium Intake

Despite advice from health professionals to cut back on sodium, salt consumption has only increased over the past 30 years, thanks to our penchant for processed foods, restaurant meals, and larger-than-ever portions. It's estimated that Canadian men consume as much as 4100 milligrams of sodium each day—more than twice the acceptable intake. Women consume roughly 2500 milligrams of sodium each day.

Aim to limit your daily sodium intake to no more than 2300 milligrams. But simply setting aside the salt shaker won't put much of a dent in your salt intake. That's because the vast majority of salt we consume each day, about 77%, is hidden away in processed and restaurant foods. Only 11% of our daily sodium comes from salt that's added during cooking and while eating. The remainder occurs naturally in foods such as milk, shellfish, and tap water.

Some of the worst sodium culprits are soups, canned vegetables, frozen dinners, processed meats, and snack foods. For instance, 1 cup (250 ml) of soup serves 500 to 1300 milligrams of sodium, depending on the brand. Frozen dinners can deliver anywhere from 400 to 1600 milligrams of sodium per serving. Breads, baked goods, and breakfast cereals also harbour sodium. Two slices of whole-wheat bread will add about 400 milligrams of sodium to your meal. And the bigger the slice of bread, the more sodium you'll consume. Restaurant meals also deliver a hefty dose of salt, especially breakfasts, Chinese entrees, and deli sandwiches.

The major risk of a high-salt diet is elevated blood pressure, a risk factor for heart attack, stroke, and kidney disease. Studies show that, on average, blood pressure rises progressively with increasing sodium intakes. People with high blood pressure, diabetes, and chronic kidney disease, as well as African Americans and older adults, are more sensitive than others to the blood pressure–raising effects of sodium. Studies show that cutting back on sodium can lower blood pressure in people with hypertension. And if you don't have hypertension, consuming less sodium can reduce your risk for developing the condition.

Sodium is added to food as sodium chloride (table salt), monosodium glutamate (MSG), sodium nitrite, sodium bicarbonate, and sodium benzoate. However, sources of sodium other than sodium chloride may have a lesser effect on blood pressure. In addition to enhancing flavour, sodium plays an important role in many foods. It's added to help control the growth of bacteria and moulds, to preserve texture, and to extend shelf life.

How Much Sodium Do You Need?

We do need some sodium for good health, but a lot less than we are currently consuming. In the body, sodium is needed to regulate fluid balance and blood pressure, and it keeps muscles and nerves working properly. People under the age of 50 need 1500 milligrams of sodium per day, people aged 50 to 70 need 1300 milligrams, and those over 70 need 1200 milligrams. Endurance athletes, such as marathoners, need more sodium to cover sweat losses that occur during exercise. The daily upper limit of sodium for adults is 2300 milligrams. Sodium sensitive individuals should limit their daily intake to less than 2300 milligrams.

The following tips will help you reduce your intake of sodium:

- Read the Nutrition Facts box on packaged foods. Sodium levels vary widely across different brands of like products. Foods with a % daily value of 5% or less are low in sodium. (The daily value for sodium is set at 2400 milligrams.)

- Pay attention to portion size. Sodium numbers on a nutrition label will underestimate your intake if you consume more than the serving size indicated.

- Limit your intake of processed meats such as bologna, ham, sausage, hot dogs, bacon, deli meats, and smoked salmon.

- Limit your use of bouillon cubes, soy sauce, Worcestershire sauce, and barbeque sauce.

- Rely less on convenience foods such as canned soups, frozen dinners, and packaged rice and pasta mixes.

- Choose pre-made entrees or frozen dinners that contain no more than 200 milligrams of sodium per 100 calories.

- When possible, choose lower sodium products. Many sodium-reduced brands contain 25% less sodium than the original version and some, such as V8 juice, contain 75% less. If you can't find low-salt products in your supermarket, ask your grocer to stock them.

- Substitute herbs and spices for salt when cooking—or try garlic, lemon juice, salsa, onion, and vinegar.

- Remove the salt shaker from the table to break the habit of salting food at the table. Every little bit counts.

Drink Plenty of Water

I can't think of any weight-loss plan that doesn't espouse "drinks lots of water" as part of its mantra. That's good advice, but not for the reasons you might think. There's a common misconception that drinking at least eight glasses of water each day helps flush fat out of your system. When losing weight, your body does not need extra water to break down body fat. You do, however, need to drink enough water to stay adequately hydrated. Your body needs water for transporting nutrients and wastes, regulating its temperature, and cushioning joints and tissues. Water may keep you healthy in other ways, too. Research suggests that drinking adequate water may guard against kidney stones, constipation, colon cancer, bladder cancer, and possibly even heart disease.

There are, however, a couple of ways in which drinking water might support your weight-loss efforts. Sometimes people confuse thirst with hunger. They reach for food when what their body really needs is water. Although there's little proof that thirst causes feelings of hunger, there is one reason why some people might confuse thirst with hunger: These sensations tend to occur together, around meal-times, especially since most people drink fluids with their meals. So the next time you feel hungry, ask yourself if your stomach really does feel empty or if you possibly could be thirsty?

There is some scientific evidence to suggest that drinking water might help you lose weight faster. One small study, conducted among men and women who were not overweight, found that drinking about 2 cups (500 ml) of water increased the subject's metabolic rate by 30%. (Your metabolic rate is the rate at which your body burns calories.) This increase occurred within 10 minutes of drinking the water. The researchers estimated that drinking 8 cups (2 litres) of water each day would help your body burn an extra 95 calories.[3]

In February 2004, the National Academy of Sciences released the first ever recommended intakes for water. Healthy, sedentary women who live in temperate climates need to drink 9 cups (2.2 litres) of water each day, while men need 13 cups (3 litres). You need to drink more water if you engage in moderate or vigorous exercise and even more if you work out in hot, humid weather. Active people who are exposed to hot weather can have daily water requirements of 24 to 32 cups (6 to 8 litres) or more per day.

The good news is that you don't have to drink 9 cups (2.2 litres) of water on top of everything else you drink. That's because, with the exception of alcoholic beverages, *all beverages* count toward your daily water recommendations. (Alcoholic beverages cause your kidneys to excrete more water and can contribute to dehydration.) These guidelines throw cold water on the notion that caffeinated beverages contribute to dehydration. If you're not used to caffeine, drinking a cup of coffee can increase urine output for a short time afterward. But people quickly build up a tolerance to the effects of caffeine. Studies show that habitual coffee drinkers do not experience increased urination or any other sign of dehydration after drinking caffeinated beverages. The bottom line: Coffee, tea, and colas all count toward your daily water.

Under normal circumstances, most of us can trust our sense of thirst to prevent becoming dehydrated. Research shows that most people meet their hydration needs simply by drinking fluids with meals and when thirsty.

On the No-Fail Diet Food and Fitness Tracker (see Appendix 1), you'll be required to keep track of how much water you consume each day. That way you'll be sure to meet the daily targets of 9 cups (2.2 litres) for women or 13 cups (3 litres) for men.

Limit Your Alcohol Intake

No doubt you've heard that a moderate intake of alcohol—one to two drinks per day—is good for your heart. Whether it's from wine, beer, or spirits, alcohol raises the level of HDL (good) cholesterol, and it may reduce blood clotting. There's also evidence that antioxidants found in wine, especially red wine, may help prevent LDL (bad) cholesterol particles from sticking to your artery walls. Keep in mind, however, that the heart-healthy effects of alcohol are most apparent in people over the age of 50 and in those with more than one risk factor for heart disease.

When it comes to cancer prevention, alcohol is definitely not a friend. Based on a comprehensive review of study findings linking alcoholic beverages to the development of many types of cancer, the experts recommend that we do not drink alcohol. Alcohol may make cells in the body more vulnerable to the effects of carcinogens or it may enhance the liver's processing of these substances. Alcohol may also inhibit the ability of cells to repair faulty genes. Finally, alcohol may increase levels of certain hormones that influence the development of cancer.

Drinking alcohol can slow down your rate of weight loss. Studies suggest that people who are overweight gain weight more easily when they drink alcohol. Alcohol does not contain fat, but it is packed with calories. One gram of alcohol (there are 14 of them in a 5 oz/150 ml glass of wine) delivers 7 calories. That's almost double the 4 calories found in 1 gram of protein. And when you add in mixers such as fruit juice or soft drinks, the calories can really add up. What's more, most studies show that people don't compensate for extra alcohol calories by eating less food. In fact, you might be tempted to eat more when you've had a few drinks. Alcohol reduces your inhibitions and general awareness of how much you're eating. Drinking on an empty stomach can also trigger food cravings.

Alcoholic beverages are not banned in the No-Fail Diet. After all, the eating plan you are about to embark on has to be a plan for life. So it doesn't make sense for me to tell you to avoid drinking a glass of wine or a cocktail. But I will tell you to keep your intake of alcoholic beverages to a minimum, and when you do drink, choose cocktails made with low-calorie mixes. These tips will help you limit your calorie intake from alcohol:

- If you're female, consume no more than seven alcoholic beverages per week, or no more than one per day. One drink is defined as 5 ounces (150 ml) of wine, 12 ounces (355 ml) of beer, or 1 1/2 ounces (45 ml) of spirits.

- If you're male, consume no more than nine alcoholic drinks per week, or two per day. But keep in mind that two drinks will add about 300 calories to your diet.

- Replace alcoholic beverages with sparkling mineral water, Clamato juice, tomato juice (a vegetable serving!), or soda water with a splash of cranberry juice.

- Dilute your calories. Order cocktails made with a calorie-free mixer, such as vodka and soda, rum and diet cola, or a white wine spritzer.

- Reserve your alcoholic beverages for meals. If you imbibe on an empty stomach, the alcohol will enter your bloodstream and make its way to your brain more quickly.

- Set your limit. Resolve ahead of time that you'll have only one or two drinks and then switch to water. Beware of waiters who keep filling your glass—it makes it hard to keep track of how much you've had to drink.

- Eliminate alcoholic beverages on evenings that you are not entertaining. Many of my clients say that their usual before-dinner drink is a habit that's easily broken. Instead, save your glass of wine or cocktail for weekends and social occasions.

Limit Your Caffeine Intake

You might have heard that drinking caffeinated beverages helps speed up weight loss. I'm afraid there is no evidence to support this notion. A few studies indicate that large amounts of caffeine (6 cups/1.5 litres of coffee a day) may slightly enhance weight loss in people who are exercising and following a low-fat diet. But there's no research to show whether this weight loss is permanent. And there is no evidence that you can lose weight by increasing your caffeine intake alone.

Some people drink coffee because they believe it suppresses their appetite, helping them eat less food. The appetite-suppressant effect of caffeine lasts only very briefly—certainly not long enough to cause weight loss. Others drink coffee while on a weight-loss diet because they've heard it speeds up calorie burning. It is true that high amounts of caffeine may increase your body's metabolism, but not enough to show a difference on the bathroom scale.

Limit your caffeine intake to 400 to 450 milligrams daily. Consuming too much caffeine can affect your health in a number of ways. Caffeine is a stimulant that increases your heart rate and blood pressure, interrupts your sleep, and causes nervousness and irritability. If you have high blood pressure, it's a good idea to keep your caffeine intake to a minimum. Research has shown that the amount of caffeine found in 2 to 3 cups (500 to 750 ml) of coffee can temporarily increase blood pressure and the stiffness of the aorta, the main artery leaving the heart. (Increased stiffness of the artery walls means that less oxygen is supplied to the heart.) Scientists speculate that this caffeine-induced stiffness of the artery wall might make high blood pressure worse and could increase the risk of heart attack or stroke in people with high blood pressure.[4]

High intakes of caffeine can also impact your bone density. That's because caffeine increases the amount of calcium you excrete in your urine. It's estimated that every 6 ounces (175 ml) of coffee leaches 48 milligrams of calcium from your bones. The negative effects of caffeine on bone health are likely most detrimental for people who are not meeting their daily calcium requirements.

Also, many caffeinated beverages, such as sugary energy drinks and Frappuccinos, are high in calories, which can cause you to gain weight if you consume them regularly.

How Much Caffeine Is Too Much?

Health Canada recommends an upper daily caffeine limit of 400 to 450 milligrams for healthy people. If you have osteoporosis, low bone density, or high blood pressure, you should aim for less caffeine. If you suffer from insomnia, I recommend that you gradually eliminate caffeine from your diet over a period of 3 weeks. Use the list below to help keep your caffeine intake under 450 milligrams per day.

Caffeine Content of Selected Beverages, Foods, and Medications (Milligrams)

Beverage	
Coffee, decaffeinated, 8 oz (250 ml)	4
Coffee, instant, 8 oz (250 ml)	80–120
Coffee, filter drip, 8 oz (250 ml)	110–180
Coffee, filter, Starbucks, grande, 16 oz (500 ml)	400
Coffee, filter, Starbucks, short, 8 oz (250 ml)	200
Cola, regular, 12 oz (355 ml)	35
Cola, diet, 12 oz (355 ml)	46
Espresso, 2 oz (60 ml)	90–100
Tea, black, 8 oz (250 ml)	46
Tea, green, 8 oz (250 ml)	33
Snacks	
Dark chocolate, 1 oz (30 g)	20
Milk chocolate, 1 oz (30 g)	6
Chocolate cake, 1 slice	20–30
Chocolate milk, 1 cup (250 ml)	8
Coffee-flavoured ice cream, Haagen-Dazs, 1/2 cup (125 ml)	24
Medication	
Excedrin, 2 pills	130
Anacin, 2 pills	64
Midol, 2 pills	64

You've learned how the four key factors of the No-Fail Diet— meal timing, protein at meals, portion size, and tracking—can help you succeed at weight loss. You've read how being physically active can enhance your weight-loss progress and help prevent you from regaining your weight once you've lost it. And in this chapter, I've explained to you the rationale behind your food choices on the No-Fail Diet, nutrition guidelines that will ensure you and your family eat healthfully while you're losing weight and for years to come. It's time to learn how to follow the No-Fail Diet.

4

The No-Fail Diet for Permanent Weight Loss

The No-Fail Diet is designed to help you lose weight and keep those pounds off for good. The meal plans and recipes that follow are designed to help you maximize your intake of nutrients that can enhance your health, energy level, and overall feeling of well-being. The meals you will eat while following the No-Fail Diet are meals that the whole family can enjoy. Just because you're losing weight doesn't mean that you need to prepare a different meal for the rest of your family. The No-Fail Diet's meal plans and recipes provide an opportunity for everyone at the table to eat healthfully. Remember: The No-Fail Diet is *not* a fad diet. Rather, it's a template for healthy eating that you can follow for the rest of your life to help you stay trim and healthy.

The No-Fail Diet is divided into three phases:

1. Phase 1 involves an optional 2-Week Quick Start meal plan. This phase is suited for people who want to follow a strict plan, for a short period, in order to see results and feel in control of their eating habits.

2. Phase 2 constitutes the bulk of the No-Fail Diet. The Phase 2 meal plan is what you will follow for 10 weeks (or 12 weeks if you opt to skip Phase 1) to achieve your weight-loss goal. If you need to follow the Phase 2 meal plan for a longer period to achieve your weight loss goal, that's perfectly fine.

3. Phase 3 teaches you how to eat to maintain your new weight over the long term.

Applying the Four Factors of the No-Fail Diet

Let's take a minute to review the four principles that are inherent to the No-Fail Diet. Applying these four principles each day will help you feel full longer after eating, have more energy during the day, and stay motivated while losing weight. Here's a quick recap:

1. *The timing factor.* You should eat every 3 to 4 hours during the day to keep your blood sugar (energy) level stable and to prevent you from becoming overly hungry at meals. If you allow yourself to get too hungry you'll be more likely to overeat. You'll notice that morning and afternoon snacks are included on the No-Fail Diet meal plans. In all likelihood, you will need to eat a snack between lunch and dinner, but depending on how many hours pass between breakfast and lunch, a morning snack might not be necessary.

2. *The protein factor.* On the No-Fail Diet, you will eat a source of protein with every meal and most snacks to help slow digestion and keep you satisfied longer after eating. On the meal plans below, you will find high-protein food and meals and snacks such as lean meat, poultry, fish, eggs, soy, legumes, nuts, milk, yogurt, or part-skim cheese.

3. *The portion-size factor.* At each meal, you will be required to size up your portions by one of three methods: 1) measuring your food with measuring cups or weighing on a food scale, 2) eyeballing your portion sizes by comparing foods with familiar objects, or 3) using the plate model when portioning foods on your plate. (All three methods are described in detail on pages 14 to 16, Chapter 1.) Once you get into the habit of monitoring the size of your food portions, it will be second nature.

4. *The tracking factor.* While following the No-Fail Diet you will keep tabs on your daily food intake and activity by keeping a journal. You'll find a Daily Food and Activity Tracker on page 337 in Appendix 1. You will also track your weight once a week and your body measurements monthly. Tracking your progress helps motivate you to keep going, and it highlights any areas in your food or exercise habits that might need improving.

The No-Fail Diet Food Groups and Serving Sizes

The meal plans that follow for Phases 1 and 2 incorporate foods from the food groups outlined below. Within each food group you will find foods low in saturated fat, refined sugars, and sodium, and high in fibre, vitamins, and minerals.

Your meal plan will indicate how many servings from each food group you need to eat each day and how you should combine them to maximize your feeling of energy. The portion size for 1 serving is listed beside each food. Serving sizes are measured *after* cooking, not before.

Protein Foods

	1 Serving Equals
Meat, Poultry, Fish, and Seafood	
Lean beef (tenderloin, sirloin, inside round, eye of round, extra-lean ground)	1 oz (30 g)
Lean pork (tenderloin, centre cut chops, lean ham, peameal bacon)	1 oz (30 g)
Veal (sirloin, loin chop, ground)	1 oz (30 g)
Chicken (skinless breast meat, extra-lean ground)	1 oz (30 g)
Turkey (skinless white or dark meat, extra-lean ground)	1 oz (30 g)
Fish, all types	1 oz (30 g)
Mussels	3 medium
Sardines, Atlantic, canned, 3 inches (7.5 cm)	2
Scallops, sea or bay	7 small or 3 large
Shrimp, large	5 (1 oz/30 g)
Oysters, raw or broiled	7 medium
Eggs and Cheese	
Egg, large, whole	1
Egg whites	2
Egg whites, liquid	1/4 cup (50 ml)
Cheese, hard, lower fat (less than 20% MF*)	1 oz (30 g)
Cheese string, part-skim	1
Cottage cheese, 1% MF or fat-free	1/4 cup (50 ml)

Vegetarian Protein Choices

Beans, cooked (black beans, chickpeas, kidney beans, navy beans, soybeans)	1/3 cup (75 ml)
Lentils, cooked	1/3 cup (75 ml)
Soy burger, 2 1/2 oz (75 g)	1/2
Soy ground round	1/4 cup (50 ml)
Soy hot dog, 1 3/4 oz (52 g)	1/2
Soy nuts, roasted	2 tbsp (25 ml)
Tempeh, cooked	1/3 cup (75 ml)
Textured soy protein (TVP), dry	3 tbsp (50 ml)
Tofu, extra-firm, chopped	1/4 cup (50 ml)

Milk and Milk Alternatives

	1 Serving Equals
Dairy	
Milk, 1% MF or skim	1 cup (250 ml)
Milk, powdered, skim	1/3 cup (75 ml)
Milk, evaporated, skim	1/2 cup (125 ml)
Yogurt, plain, 1% MF or skim	1 cup (250 ml)
Yogurt, flavoured or fruit bottom, 1% MF or skim	3/4 cup (175 ml or 175 g container)
Non-Dairy	
Rice beverage, plain, calcium-enriched	1 cup (250 ml)
Soy beverage, plain, calcium-enriched	1 cup (250 ml)

Starchy Foods

	1 Serving Equals
Breads (choose a whole grain bread most often)	
Bread	1 slice (30 g)
Bagel, small	1/2 (30 g)
Bagel, regular size	1/4 (1 oz/30 g)
Bun (kaiser roll, hamburger roll)	1/2
English muffin	1/2
Pita pocket, 6 inch (15 cm)	1/2 (1 oz/30 g)
Tortilla, soft, 6 inch (15 cm)	1
Tortilla, soft, 10 inch (25 cm)	1/2

Cereals (choose whole grain cereals most often)

Cold cereal, dry flake (e.g., Bran Flakes, Cheerios, Shreddies, Shredded Wheat Spoon Size)	3/4 cup (175 ml)
Cold cereal, denser, flake (e.g., Kashi Golean, Nature's Path Flax Plus, Nature's Path Optimum)	1/2 cup (125 ml)
Cold cereal, 100% bran	1/2 cup (125 ml)
Granola	1/4 cup (50 ml)
Kellogg's All-Bran Buds	1/3 cup (75 ml)
Oats, dry	1/4 cup (50 ml)
Oatmeal, cooked	1/2 cup (125 ml)
Oatmeal, instant, unflavoured	1 pouch
Shredded Wheat	1 biscuit

Crackers

Finn Crisp crackers	5 slices
Rice cakes, brown	2
Rice crackers, small	10
Soda crackers, whole-wheat	7
Ryvita crispbread	3 slices
Wasa crackers	1 1/2 slices

Grains and Potatoes

Barley or bulgur, cooked	1/3 cup (75 ml)
Corn	1/2 cup (125 ml) or 1/2 cob
Couscous, cooked	1/3 cup (75 ml)
Pasta, whole-wheat, cooked	1/2 cup (125 ml)
Potato, new or yellow flesh	1/2 medium or 1/2 cup (125 ml)
Potato, sweet	1/2 medium or 1/2 cup (125 ml)
Quinoa, cooked	1/3 cup (75 ml)
Rice, brown or wild, cooked	1/3 cup (75 ml)

Other Starchy Foods

Granola bar, low-fat, small (approximately 90 calories)	1
Muffins, very small, low-fat, whole-grain	1/2
Popcorn, air popped or low-fat microwave	3 cups (750 ml)
Soup, broth based with potato, rice, or pasta	1 cup (250 ml)

Fruit

	1 Serving Equals
Fresh Fruit	
Apple	1 medium
Apricots	4

Banana	1 small
Blackberries	1 cup (250 ml)
Blueberries	1 cup (250 ml)
Cantaloupe or honeydew	1/2 small or 1 cup (250 ml) cubes
Figs	2 small
Fruit, canned, packed in water or juice	1 cup (250 ml)
Grapefruit	1 small
Grapes	40 or 1 cup (250 ml)
Kiwi	1 medium
Mango	1/2 medium
Nectarine	1 medium
Orange	1 medium
Papaya	1/2 medium
Peach	1 medium
Pear	1 medium
Pineapple, fresh or canned in water or juice	3/4 cup (175 ml)
Plums	4
Raspberries	1 cup (250 ml)
Strawberries	1 1/2 cups (375 ml)
Watermelon, diced	1 1/2 cups (375 ml)
Dried Fruit	
Apricots	7 halves
Cranberries	2 tbsp (25 ml)
Dates	3
Figs	3
Prunes	4
Raisins	2 tbsp (25 ml)
Unsweetened, 100% Fruit Juices	
Apple, grapefruit, orange, pineapple	1/2 cup (125 ml)
Cranberry, grape, prune	1/3 cup (75 ml)

Vegetables

	1 Serving Equals
Aim to eat at least three different coloured vegetables each day.	1/2 cup (125 ml) cooked or raw or 1 cup (250 ml) mixed greens or 1/2 cup (125 ml) vegetable juice

Green	Yellow/Orange	Red
artichokes	butternut squash	beets
arugula	carrots	radishes

asparagus	pumpkin	radicchio
beet greens	rutabagas	red onions
broccoli	yellow peppers	red peppers
broccoflower	yellow summer squash	tomato juice
Brussels sprouts	yellow tomatoes	tomatoes
celery	winter squash	
Chinese cabbage		
collard greens		
cucumber		
endive		
green beans		
green cabbage		
green leaf lettuce	**White**	**Blue/Purple**
green pepper	cauliflower	eggplant
kale	jicama	purple cabbage
okra	kohlrabi	purple carrots
peas	mushrooms	purple endive
rapini	onions	purple peppers
romaine lettuce	parsnips	
snow peas	turnips	
spinach		
Swiss chard		
watercress		
zucchini		

Fats and Oils

	1 Serving Equals
Spreads	
Butter or non-hydrogenated margarine	1 tsp (5 ml)
Margarine, light	2 tsp (10 ml)
Cream cheese, fat-reduced	2 tbsp (25 ml)
Dressings and Oils	
Mayonnaise, regular	1 tsp (5 ml)
Mayonnaise, fat-reduced	2 tsp (10 ml)
Peanut sauce, calorie reduced	2 tbsp (25 ml)
Pesto sauce, bottled	1 1/2 tsp (7 ml)
Salad dressing, fat-reduced	4 tsp (20 ml)
Salad dressing, vinaigrette	2 tsp (10 ml)
Vegetable oil (olive, canola, flaxseed, walnut)	1 tsp (5 ml)

Other Fats	
Almonds, dry roasted	6
Goat cheese, soft, 20% MF or less	1 tbsp (15 ml)
Parmesan cheese, grated	2 tbsp (25 ml)
Peanuts, dry roasted	1 tbsp (15 ml)
Pecans, dry roasted	5 halves
Walnuts	4 halves
Avocado	1/8
Dips (hummus, tzatziki)	2 tbsp (25 ml)
Nut butter	1 1/2 tsp (7 ml)
Olives, medium	6
Seeds	1 tbsp (15 ml)
Sour cream, fat-reduced, 7% MF	2 tbsp (25 ml)

* milk fat

Water Requirements on the No-Fail Diet

You must drink water throughout the day on the No-Fail Diet to stay adequately hydrated. Drinking water with meals and between meals also helps fill your stomach and may help prevent overeating. Women need to drink 9 cups (2.2 litres) of water each day; men need to drink 13 cups (3 litres).

All beverages, with the exception of alcoholic beverages, count toward your daily water requirements. In addition to plain drinking water, your water can come from unsweetened fruit juice, vegetable juice, milk, soy milk, coffee, tea, herbal tea, and diet soft drinks. However, the majority of your daily water should come from drinking water, herbal tea, tea, and some coffee, so that you don't consume more calories than allowed on your meal plan. You will be required to record your daily water intake on the Food and Activity Tracker.

Alcoholic Beverages on the No-Fail Diet

Alcoholic beverages add calories to your diet. In Phase 1, alcoholic beverages are not allowed. In Phase 2, they must be kept to a minimum if you want to continue to lose weight. But don't worry, you are allowed to enjoy the occasional glass of wine with dinner, or when dining out. Your weight-loss plan must be realistic and one that you can comfortably live with.

You may need to reduce your current intake of alcoholic beverages, however. In Phase 2 of the No-Fail Diet, women will be allowed to have a weekly maximum of seven drinks; men will be allowed to have no more than nine. (One drink is equivalent to 5 oz/150 ml of wine, 1 1/2 oz/45 ml of spirits, and 12 oz/355 ml of light beer.) Avoid mixed drinks with fruit juice, tonic water, and sugary soft drinks, as these add unwanted calories to your diet. You will track your weekly intake of alcoholic beverages on the Food and Activity Tracker provided in Appendix 1.

If you don't drink that many drinks now, do not consider this as permission to increase your intake. If you don't drink any alcohol, or if you have only a couple of drinks each week, maintain this low intake—it's better for your weight and your health.

Nutrition Supplements on the No-Fail Diet

It's a nice notion that a balanced diet can provide you with all the vitamins and minerals you need each day. Even if you weren't reducing your calorie intake to lose weight, it can be challenging to get every nutrient you need unless you carefully plan all your food choices. If you eat on the run, skip meals, or make poor food choices, your diet is likely to come up short on a few vitamins and minerals.

Eating fewer calories in an effort to lose weight makes it challenging to consume the recommended intakes of iron, calcium, and vitamin D. Menstruating women need 18 milligrams of iron each day, an amount that can be difficult to obtain from even a 2000 calorie diet if you don't eat red meat often (3 oz/90 g of lean beef provides 3.3 milligrams of iron). If you're a female vegetarian, you need 32 milligrams, since iron from plant sources is not absorbed as well as iron from animal sources. Men and postmenopausal women need 8 milligrams of iron each day, an amount that's much easier to get from the No-Fail Diet meal plans. (Vegetarian men and postmenopausal women need 14 milligrams of iron each day.)

If you are between the ages of 19 to 50, you need 1000 milligrams of calcium each day. In food terms, that means you need to consume 3 cups (750 ml) of milk, yogurt, enriched soy milk, or enriched fruit juice every day. If you're over the age of 50, you need 1500 milligrams of calcium daily—the amount found in 5 cups (1.25 litres) of milk, yogurt, or fortified beverage. You will notice that Level 1 and Level 2 meal plans include 2 servings from the Milk and Milk Alternative food group (providing 600 milligrams of calcium). The Level 3 and Level 4 meal plans each provide 900 milligrams of calcium from 3 Milk and Milk Alternative servings. You'll get more calcium if you include in your diet part-skim cheese, canned salmon with the bones, and tofu (found in the Protein Foods group) as well as leafy green vegetables, nuts, and seeds.

To make sure all your nutrient needs are adequately covered, I recommend a multivitamin and mineral supplement every day, along with a calcium supplement.

Multivitamin and Mineral Supplements

An all-purpose one-a-day multivitamin provides your daily require-ments for most nutrients, with the exception of calcium and magne-sium. Depending on your age, a multivitamin may not supply enough iron and vitamin D. In addition to helping women meet their daily iron targets, a multivitamin and mineral supplement is an important way for adults over 50 to get vitamin B12 (as we age, out bodies become less efficient at absorbing B12 from foods). A multivitamin will also help you meet your requirements for folic acid, a B vitamin linked with protection from heart disease, breast cancer, and colon cancer.

Menstruating women should choose a formula that supplies 0.4 to 1 milligram of folic acid, 10 to 18 milligrams of iron, and 400 IU (international units) vitamin D. Postmenopausal women and men of all ages should choose a formula that supplies 0.4 to 1 milligram of folic acid, 5 to 10 milligrams of iron, and 400 IU of vitamin D.

If your doctor has told you that your iron levels are too high, or that you have hemochromatosis, choose a formula that is iron-free.

(Hemochromatosis is a disorder that causes the body to absorb too much iron from foods. The excess iron is stored in the organs, especially the liver, heart, and pancreas. Stored iron can sometimes damage these organs and lead to serious health problems.)

Calcium Supplements

IF YOU ARE 19 TO 49 YEARS OLD:

Buy a product that provides 300 to 500 milligrams of calcium. Buy a calcium supplement with added vitamin D (200 or 400 IU).

Phase 1: Take one calcium supplement daily with a meal.

Phase 2: Levels 1 and 2 (1200 and 1400 calories): Take one calcium supplement daily with a meal.

Phase 2: Levels 3 and 4 (1700 and 2000 calories): A calcium supplement is not required.

IF YOU HAVE OSTEOPENIA (LOW BONE DENSITY)
OR OSTEOPOROSIS, OR YOU ARE 50 YEARS OR OLDER:

Buy a product that provides 500 milligrams of calcium and 200 or 400 IU of vitamin D per tablet.

Phase 1: Take one calcium supplement twice daily with a meal.

Phase 2: Take one calcium supplement twice daily with a meal, regardless of what calorie level you are adhering to.

To reduce cancer risk, Canadian adults are advised to supplement their diets with 1000 IU of vitamin D in the fall and winter—and all year round if you don't expose your skin, unprotected, to sunshine in the summer months. Calculate how much vitamin D your multivitamin and calcium supplements provide. If necessary, make up the difference with a stand-alone vitamin D supplement.

Phase 1: 2-Week Quick Start on the No-Fail Diet

The No-Fail Diet begins with an optional Quick Start meal plan. This is an optional phase; it is not necessary to follow the 2-Week Quick Start meal plan. You may opt to skip Phase 1 and jump ahead to

Phase 2, outlined below. How can you decide if you should follow Phase 1, the 2-Week Quick Start? If you answer yes to one or more of the following statements, you're a good candidate:

- I need to see results quickly to stay motivated when making changes to my diet.

- My schedule and lifestyle make it relatively easy for me to follow a restrictive diet for 2 weeks.

- I find that going "cold turkey" for a short period helps me to break bad eating habits.

- I feel that I am addicted to starchy foods.

- I don't get bored easily with foods. I don't mind eating the same types of foods at meals for a short period.

Phase 1 isn't for everyone. Some people will find it easy to be restrictive with their food intake for 2 weeks, others won't. If you travel, dine out frequently, or have a busy social calendar, this phase might not work for you. And that's okay. Just move directly to Phase 2, the sustained weight-loss phase of the No-Fail Diet.

The 2-Week Quick Start meal plan is intended for people who feel they need to see results quickly in order to get and stay motivated. It's for people who need to jumpstart their weight loss. Phase 1 is a short-term plan that's easy to follow and will help break bad eating habits. Phase 1 is useful for people who find it easier to adhere to a plan if avoidance of certain foods, rather than moderation, is the operative word. Such a plan can help people eliminate cravings for starchy foods such as bread and crackers, or sugary and high-fat junk foods. If you are in control of the majority of your meals (that is, you are not required to dine out often), you shouldn't have a problem sticking to Phase 1 for 2 weeks.

Phase 1 of the No-Fail Diet is designed to be followed for 2 weeks only. The Quick Start meal plan applies the four key factors described earlier: timing, protein at meals, portion size, and tracking, and involves the No-Fail Diet food groups.

2-Week Quick Start Meal Plan

Food Group	Number of Servings per Day	
	Women	Men
Protein Foods	6	9
Starchy Foods	1 to 2	2 to 3
Milk and Milk Alternatives	2	2
Fruit	2	2
Vegetables	7	7
Fats and Oils	4	6

In Phase 1 of the No-Fail Diet, the following rules must be adhered to:

1. Starchy foods are to be eaten only with breakfast. Starchy foods are not allowed at lunch, dinner, or snacks.

2. Alcoholic beverages are not allowed.

3. No desserts or foods high in refined sugars are to be eaten (a weekly treat will be introduced in Phase 2).

4. Take one 30-minute brisk walk each day (or two 15-minute walks daily), or follow the No-Fail 12-Week Fitness Program outlined in Chapter 5.

Why so few starchy foods? In a nutshell, because these are the foods that many people tend to overeat. I call foods such as bread, pasta, rice, and starchy snack foods "risky foods" because people often complain it's difficult to keep their portion sizes small. Sometimes it's because the food just tastes so good. Many clients tell me they have trouble limiting their portion of homemade pasta and meat sauce, or they eat too many slices of pizza. Starchy snacks such as pretzels, crackers, and cereal bars can also trigger overeating because they don't fill you up. And it's easy to overeat starchy foods because big food is the norm today in restaurants, coffee shops, and grocery stores. We eat bagels the equivalent of five slices of bread, huge muffins, economy-size bags of pretzels ... the list goes on. Research shows that the more food we put in front of us, the more likely it is that we'll eat more than we need.

Phase 1 removes these temptations for you by eliminating starchy foods at lunch and dinner and at snack times. Phase 1 is *not* a low-carb diet. Rather it's a moderate-carbohydrate, moderate-protein diet that is low in fat. During the next 2 weeks, you will continue to eat healthy carbohydrate foods such as whole grains, fruit, and milk. However, I have limited your intake of starchy foods to breakfast only. If overeating carbs is a major reason why you're carrying extra weight, eliminating starchy foods at lunch, dinner, and snacks will help you kick-start weight loss. Your body will get used to eating them less often and you'll stop craving them. What's more, you'll replace these starchy foods with nutritious foods that do not trigger overeating. The Phase 1 meal plan will especially help you boost your intake of vegetables.

Phase 1 also introduces physical activity into your day. You are encouraged to follow the 12-Week Fitness Program that is detailed in Chapter 5. If you are not ready for this, you must accumulate 30 minutes of brisk walking every day. If you are short on time, you can split this into two 15-minute walks. And whenever possible, add small amounts of physical activity to your daily routine. I have outlined ways to become more active on page 43 in Chapter 2.

Because women and men differ in their calorie and protein needs, I have outlined two meal plans—one for women an another for men. You'll notice that the meal plan for men has an additional 3 servings of Protein Foods and 1 extra serving from the Starchy Foods group. This means that portion sizes of protein at lunch and dinner will be larger for men, as will their starch serving at breakfast.

Mapping Out Your Meals in Phase 1

Women

Food Group	Breakfast	Snack 1	Lunch	Snack 2	Dinner
Protein Foods			2		4
Starchy Foods	1 to 2		0		0
Milk and Milk Alternatives	1	1			
Fruit	1	1			
Vegetables			3	1	3
Fats and Oils			2	1	1

Men

Food Group	Breakfast	Snack 1	Lunch	Snack 2	Dinner
Protein Foods			3		6
Starchy Foods	2 to 3		0		0
Milk and Milk Alternatives	1	1			
Fruit	1	1			
Vegetables			3	1	3
Fats and Oils	1		2	1	2

Moving Food Servings from One Meal to Another

The meal plan above is intended to serve as a guide to help you space out your food over the course of a day. I have mapped out your food servings at meals to keep you feeling full and to help keep your blood sugar level stable longer after eating. This will reduce the likelihood of you feeling hungry and low in energy. However, your meal plan should be flexible enough so that you can add variety to meals. You may make the following changes, if you wish:

- You may move 1 Protein Food serving from dinner to breakfast. For example, you might decide you would like to have one boiled egg with your slice of toast, or 1/4 cup (50 ml) low-fat cottage cheese on your fruit salad.

- You may move your servings of Fats and Oils from one meal to another, or from one meal to a snack. For example, if you'd like to have 1 1/2 teaspoons (7 ml) of peanut butter on your whole-grain toast at breakfast, you may take 1 Fats and Oils serving from either lunch or dinner. (The meal plan for men includes 1 Fats and Oils serving at breakfast. If you do not use it at this meal, feel free to move it to another meal or snack.)

Phase 1 Meal Ideas

The meal ideas below provide the recommended serving sizes for women. If you are a male, add 1 or 2 Starchy Food servings at breakfast, 1 Protein Food serving at lunch, and 2 Protein Food servings at dinner, referring to the list of food groups on page 76.

Phase 1 Breakfasts

You can choose any of the following breakfasts on Phase 1 of the No-Fail Diet. The meals below all provide 1 Starchy Food serving, 1 Milk and Milk Alternatives serving, and 1 Fruit serving. (Remember, you may move 1 Protein Food serving from dinner to breakfast. You may also move 1 Fats and Oils serving from lunch or dinner to breakfast, if desired.)

1. High-fibre cereal with yogurt and fruit
    1/2 cup (125 ml) 100% bran cereal (e.g., Kellogg's All-Bran Original, PC Blue Menu Fibre First)
    3/4 cup (175 ml or 175 g container) low-fat plain or sugar-free yogurt
    1 cup (250 ml) blueberries
    Water: tea, coffee, plain water

2. Whole-grain cereal with milk and juice
    3/4 cup (175 ml) whole-grain flake cereal
    1 cup (250 ml) skim, 1% milk fat (MF), or enriched soy milk (unflavoured)
    1/2 cup (125 ml) unsweetened orange or grapefruit juice
    Water: tea, coffee, plain water

3. Hot cereal with yogurt and dried fruit
    1/2 cup (125 ml) cooked oatmeal or Red River cereal
    3/4 cup (175 ml or 175 g container) low-fat plain or sugar-free vanilla-flavoured yogurt
    2 tbsp (25 ml) raisins or dried cranberries
    Water: tea, coffee, plain water

4. Whole-grain toast with fruit salad and café latte
    1 slice whole-grain toast
    Sugar-reduced fruit spread
    1 cup (250 ml) mixed fruit salad
    Latte made with 1 cup (250 ml) skim, 1% MF, or enriched plain soy milk

5. Whole-grain pancake with fruit and yogurt
    1 small whole-wheat pancake topped with 1/2 cup (125 ml) sugar-free vanilla yogurt, 1/2 cup (125 ml) berries, and 1/2 small banana, sliced
    1 cup (250 ml) coffee or tea with up to 1/2 cup (125 ml) skim, 1% MF, or enriched plain soy milk
    Water: tea, coffee, plain water

Phase 1 Lunches

Both your lunch and dinner meals consist of Protein Foods, Vegetables, and healthy Fats and Oils. The only difference between these two meals is the portion size of Protein Foods. At lunch you will have 2 servings of Protein Foods and at dinner you will have 4 servings (women). To help you feel satisfied, fill your plate with at least 3 servings of vegetables (1 1/2 cups/375 ml). Use the following meal ideas to get you started (feel free to use any of the marinade recipes from Chapter 7 to spice up your meals).

1. Chef's Salad

    Large green salad with leafy greens and chopped vegetables as desired

    1/2 184 g can tuna or 2 hard-cooked eggs OR 1 hard-cooked egg and 1 oz (30 g) part-skim cheese

    4 walnut halves

    2 tsp (10 ml) salad dressing

    Water

2. Veggie omelet with salad

    Make your omelet using 1 whole egg and 2 egg whites (use non-stick cooking spray)

    Add sliced mushrooms, chopped red bell pepper, and baby spinach leaves

    Mixed greens with 1 tbsp (15 ml) sunflower seeds

    2 tsp (10 ml) salad dressing

    Water

3. Cottage cheese salad

    Mix 1/2 cup (125 ml) 1% MF cottage cheese with 1/2 chopped green pepper and 1 chopped tomato; serve on a bed of greens

    Sprinkle with 2 tbsp (25 ml) toasted pine nuts or sunflower seeds

    Water

4. Italian-style vegetable soup with legumes

    1 1/2 cups (375 ml) hearty vegetable soup (homemade or store bought)

    Add 2/3 cup (150 ml) lentils or kidney beans to soup

    Sprinkle with 1 tbsp (15 ml) grated Parmesan cheese

    Mixed greens with 2 tsp (10 ml) salad dressing

    Water

5. Hot and sour soup with tofu and veggies

   1 1/2 cups (375 ml) hot and sour soup*

   Add 1/2 cup (125 ml) chopped extra-firm tofu and 1 cup (250 ml) chopped kale or spinach

   On the side: 1/2 cup (125 ml) raw vegetable sticks with 2 tbsp (25 ml) hummus

   Water

   * When shopping for hot and sour soup at the grocery store, look for fresh varieties sold in mason jars (e.g., Soup's On, Summer Fresh, Neil's Kitchen).

6. Veggie burger with greens

   1 soy-based burger, grilled

   2 cups (500 ml) mixed greens with 1/8 avocado, sliced

   2 tsp (10 ml) salad dressing

   Water

7. Leftovers from dinner

   2 oz (60 g) lean meat, chicken, or salmon

   1 1/2 cups (375 ml) stir-fried, steamed, or grilled vegetables

   2 tsp (10 ml) extra-virgin olive oil

   Water

Phase 1 Dinners

Making a dinner consisting only of protein and vegetables doesn't involve a lot of thinking. It's a cinch to grill a chicken breast or salmon fillet and serve it with a medley of steamed veggies. Or throw a can of tuna over a bed of greens. It's even easy to stir-fry some lean beef or tofu with a bunch of vegetables. Ease of meal planning is the upside. But meals without starchy foods can be boring if you do the same old meat-and-veggies routine. I encourage you to add a variety of tastes to your dinners. Try one or more of the meal ideas below to help prevent boredom. You'll find these recipes, plus many more, in Chapter 7.

1. Rosemary Mustard Chicken (recipe on page 310)

   Serve with 1 to 1 1/2 cups (250 to 375 ml) steamed, stir-fried, or grilled vegetables

   1 cup (250 ml) mixed greens

   4 tsp (20 ml) regular salad dressing

2. Hoisin-Brushed Salmon

    Brush a 4 oz (120 g) salmon fillet with 1 to 2 tbsp (15 to 25 ml) hoisin sauce*

    Bake at 450°F (230°C) for 10 minutes per inch of thickness

    Serve with 1 to 1 1/2 cups (250 to 375 ml) steamed, stir-fried, or grilled vegetables

    1 cup (250 ml) mixed greens

    2 tsp (10 ml) regular salad dressing

    * Hoisin sauce is sold in the ethnic food section of most grocery stores.

3. Sesame Tofu Stir-Fry (recipe on page 322)

4. Tomato Herb Fish (recipe on page 300)

    1 large grilled portobello mushroom (Drizzle with 1 tsp/5 ml olive oil and a dash of balsamic vinegar and grill for 12 to 15 minutes.)

    Serve with 1 to 1 1/2 cups (250 to 375 ml) of your favourite steamed vegetables

5. Honey Glazed Pork Tenderloin (recipe on page 307)

    1 cup (250 ml) eggplant and zucchini, drizzled with 1 tsp (5 ml) oil and grilled for 15 to 20 minutes

6. Spaghetti Squash Pasta (recipe on page 311)

    2 cups (500 ml) mixed greens with 4 tsp (20 ml) regular salad dressing

7. Mango Chutney Salmon (see recipe on page 295)

    1 cup (250 ml) spinach, steamed and drizzled with 1 tsp (5 ml) sesame oil

    1 cup (250 ml) mixed greens with 2 tsp (10 ml) regular salad dressing

Snacks in Phase 1

You must eat every 3 to 4 hours, so that means you will need to eat midday snacks: one between breakfast and lunch, and another between lunch and dinner. You may not need to eat both snacks. For example, if you eat breakfast at 8:00 or 8:30 A.M. and lunch at noon, you can skip the morning snack if you like. But snacks should always be eaten when your meals are spaced more than 4 hours apart. *If you don't feel the need for one of your snacks, move those food servings to your other snack or a meal.*

I have given you 1 Fruit serving, 1 Milk serving, 1 Vegetable serving, and 1 Fat serving to include in your snacks. You can mix these up as you wish when planning your snacks. Here are a few snack suggestions:

FOR A SNACK THAT PROVIDES 1 FRUIT + 1 MILK SERVING, CHOOSE ONE OF:

- 3/4 cup (175 ml or 175 g container) low-fat plain or sugar-free yogurt + 1 medium fruit or 1 cup (250 ml) berries
- Homemade smoothie (in the blender, whirl together 1 cup/ 250 ml low-fat milk or soy milk with 1/2 cup/125 ml frozen berries and 1/2 small banana)
- 1 cup (250 ml) calcium-fortified soy milk (unflavoured) + 1 apple or small banana

FOR A SNACK THAT PROVIDES 1 VEGETABLE AND 1 FAT SERVING, CHOOSE ONE OF:

- 1 cup (250 ml) vegetable or tomato juice + 6 plain, unsalted almonds
- 1/2 cup (125 ml) raw vegetables + 2 tbsp (25 ml) hummus
- 1/2 cup (125 ml) baby carrots + 6 medium olives
- 6 celery sticks + 2 tbsp (25 ml) fat-reduced cream cheese

FOR A SNACK THAT PROVIDES 1 FRUIT + 1 FAT SERVING, CHOOSE ONE OF:

- 1 sliced apple + 1 1/2 tsp (7 ml) peanut butter
- 1 sliced pear + 1 tbsp (15 ml) soft goat cheese (20% MF or less)
- 1 cup (250 ml) fruit salad + 1 tbsp (15 ml) sunflower seeds
- 7 dried apricot halves + 4 walnut halves (or 6 whole almonds)

Phase 2: Sustaining Weight Loss on the No-Fail Diet, Weeks 3 to 12

If you decide not to follow Phase 1, then Phase 2 is your starting point. If you followed Phase 1 for 2 weeks, you are now ready to move to an eating plan that will serve you well as you continue to lose weight—and over the long term. I do not believe that there is one diet for everyone. We are all different and, as such, have unique calorie and nutrient needs. That's why I have outlined four meal plans, each corresponding to a different calorie level.

Which meal plan you choose will depend on your gender (men need more calories than women), your current weight (heavier bodies require more calories), and your activity level. If you are very active, you will generally need to eat more calories to sustain your exercise program. Exercising regularly allows you to enjoy more food while you're losing weight. Now that you have become familiar with the food groups and serving sizes, here are the meal plans that you will follow for the next 10 weeks.

The No-Fail Diet Meal Plans

Food Group	Level 1 1200 calories	Level 2 1400 calories	Level 3 1700 calories	Level 4 2000 calories
		Number of Servings per Day		
Protein Foods	5	6	7	9
Starchy Foods	4	5	6	7
Milk and Milk Alternatives	2	2	3	3
Fruit	2	2	3	3
Vegetables	4	4	4	4
Fats and Oils	3	4	4	6

Which Calorie Level Is Right for You?

Basically, if you eat 500 fewer calories than you normally do each day, you should lose about 1 pound (0.5 kg) per week, since 1 pound (0.5 kg) of body fat is equivalent to 3500 calories. If you eat 1000 fewer calories each day, you'll lose about 2 pounds (0.9 kg) each week. But most people don't know how many calories they typically consume each day. Ultimately, which meal plan you choose comes down to your activity level, your height, your sex, and how many pounds you'd like to lose each week. Use the following guidelines to decide which meal plan is best for you:

• In general, most women should choose Level 1 or Level 2. If you are sedentary (and you don't plan to increase your activity level while losing weight), choose Level 1, 1200 calories.

However, if you are taller than the average woman (your height is 65 inches/162.5 cm or taller), consider opting for Level 2, 1400 calories.

- If you are an active female (you exercise for 30 to 60 minutes 3 or 4 days per week) or you plan to become active on the No-Fail Diet, choose Level 2, 1400 calories.

- If you are a very active female (you exercise for 1 hour or more, most days of the week), choose Level 3, 1700 calories.

- If you are a sedentary man (and you don't plan to add daily physical activity), choose Level 3, 1700 calories. If you are taller than the average male (your height is 71 inches/177.5 cm or taller), choose Level 4, 2000 calories.

- If you are a physically active male (you exercise for 30 to 60 minutes 3 or more days per week), choose Level 4, 2000 calories.

Keep in mind that you can always change your calorie level at any time on the No-Fail Diet. For example, if you start at Level 1 (1200 calories) and find that you're losing more than 2 pounds (0.9 kg) each week, switch to Level 2, the 1400 calorie meal plan. Conversely, if after following the Level 3 meal plan (1700 calories) you find you're losing about 1 pound (0.5 kg) per week and would prefer to lose weight a little faster, drop your daily calorie intake to 1400 (Level 2).

Using the Meal Plans

Each meal plan is designed to help you eat a well-balanced diet that includes foods from all six food groups. The meal plans will help you reduce your intake of saturated and trans fats and increase your intake of fibre, vitamins, minerals, and protective plant chemicals (phytochemicals). Once you've chosen which meal plan you will follow, you need to map out your daily food servings over the course of the day, in order to keep you feeling satisfied and energetic. That's where the timing factor and protein factor come into play. In the example below, I have divided the recommended servings of food groups among meals and snacks. You will notice that I have included a protein-rich food at each meal and snack.

Level 1: 1200 calories

	Breakfast	Lunch	Dinner	Snack(s)
Protein Foods		2	3	
Starchy Foods	1	2	1	
Milk and Milk Alternatives	1			1
Fruit	1			1
Vegetables		1	2	1
Fats and Oils		1	1	1

Level 2: 1400 calories

	Breakfast	Lunch	Dinner	Snack(s)
Protein Foods		3	3	
Starchy Foods	1	2	2	
Milk and Milk Alternatives	1			1
Fruit	1			1
Vegetables		1	2	1
Fats and Oils	1	1	1	1

Level 3: 1700 calories

	Breakfast	Lunch	Dinner	Snack(s)
Protein Foods		3	4	
Starchy Foods	2	2	2	
Milk and Milk Alternatives	1	1		1
Fruit	1			2
Vegetables		1	2	1
Fats and Oils	1	1	1	1

Level 4: 2000 calories

	Breakfast	Lunch	Dinner	Snack(s)
Protein Foods		4	5	
Starchy Foods	2	2	3	
Milk and Milk Alternatives	1	1		1
Fruit	1			2
Vegetables		1	2	1
Fats and Oils	1	2	2	1

Moving Food Servings from One Meal to Another

The meal plan above is intended to serve as a guideline to help you space out your food over the course of a day. The way I have mapped out the food servings at meals is designed to help you feel fuller at meals and to help keep your blood sugar level stable longer after eating. Eating the right combinations of food groups at meals and snacks, at regular intervals during the day, will reduce the likelihood that you'll feel hungry and be low in energy.

The meal plans suggested above are not set in stone. Your meal plan should be flexible, so you may make the following changes, if you wish:

- You may move 1 Starchy Food serving from one meal to another. I typically don't recommend eating starchy foods as midday snacks because many don't keep you feeling satisfied to the same degree that fruit, dairy, or other foods with protein do. However, starchy foods with a low glycemic index (GI) are an exception. Low GI starchy foods such as plain popcorn, Ryvita crackers, and Finn Crisp crackers are more slowly digested than refined (white) starchy foods. If, on occasion, you would like to move 1 Starchy Food serving from a meal to your snack, you may do so. Just make sure to replace that Starchy Food serving in the meal with the food you will not be eating for your snack (e.g., fruit, yogurt, milk, soy milk, veggies, and hummus).

- With the exception of breakfast, you may move 1 Milk and Milk Alternative serving from lunch to dinner (this applies to the 1700 and 2000 calorie meal plan only).

- You may move 1 Protein Food serving from lunch or dinner to breakfast.

- You may move your servings of Fats and Oils from one meal to another, or from one meal to a snack. For example, if you'd like to have peanut butter on your whole-grain toast at breakfast, feel free to use 1 Fat serving from lunch or dinner.

- You may add more vegetables to any meal you like. With the exception of green peas, which are relatively high in calories, vegetables are unlimited. Each meal plan includes a minimum of 4 daily vegetable servings.

- You may eliminate the Starchy Food servings at dinner if you like. If you do so, increase your intake of Protein Foods by 2 servings and add more vegetables to your meal.

Because your meal plan is designed to prevent you from feeling hungry between meals, or overly hungry before meals, keep the following rules in mind when making changes to your basic meal plan:

- Do not skip meals. Always eat three meals plus at least one midday snack.

- Breakfast must always include at least 1 protein-rich food serving, from Milk and Milk Alternatives or Protein Foods.

- Lunch and dinner must always include servings from the Protein Foods group.

- While it's okay to move a few food servings from lunch to dinner in anticipation of a big meal, it is not okay to skip lunch entirely to save calories for a large dinner. You'll just wind up feeling ravenous before dinner, making you far more inclined to overeat.

What Kind of Snacks Can You Eat?

It's easy to visualize what lunch or dinner might be just by looking at the allotted number of food servings on your meal plan. For example, a lunch consisting of 3 Protein Food servings and 2 Starchy Food servings might be a sandwich made with 3 ounces (90 g) of turkey and two slices of whole-grain bread, or it might be 3/4 cup (175 ml) stir-fried tofu on 2/3 cup (150 ml) brown rice. But it's not always easy to visualize snacks. Here are a few suggested snacks, and the food group servings they count as:

Snack	Counts as (Food Group Servings) ...
1 apple and 1 part-skim cheese string	1 Fruit, 1 Protein Food
3/4 cup (175 ml or 175 g container) yogurt with 1/2 cup (125 ml) fruit	1 Milk and Milk Alternative, 1/2 Fruit
1 cup grapes + 6 plain almonds	1 Fruit, 1 Fat and Oil
1 to 1 1/2 cups (250 to 375 ml) smoothie (1 cup/250 ml milk, 1/2 banana, 1/2 cup/125 ml berries)	1 Fruit, 1 Milk and Milk Alternative

3 cups (750 ml) plain popcorn with 1 tsp (5 ml) margarine	1 Starchy Food, 1 Fat and Oil
1 energy bar (e.g., Clif Luna Bar or PowerBar Pria)	1 Starchy Food, 1 Protein Food
1 medium (12 oz/375 ml) skim or soy latte	1 Milk and Milk Alternative
1 cup (250 ml) fruit salad with 1/4 cup (50 ml) cottage cheese	1 Fruit, 1 Protein Food

You'll find these and other snacks, along with breakfast, lunch, and dinner ideas, in the No-Fail Diet Menu Plans, outlined in Chapter 6.

Plan a Weekly Splurge in Phase 2

To be successful at losing weight, it's important that you do not feel deprived. Swearing off your favourite food will ultimately make you feel miserable. As soon as you put a food on a forbidden list, it becomes more desirable. When you're stressed or bored, you're more likely to crave what's taboo, a feeling that can lead to bingeing. Then the diet mentality sets in: You scold yourself for breaking your diet and resolve to start again tomorrow.

That's why I do not recommend that you completely banish your favourite treats, be it cookies, cake, ice cream, chocolate, french fries, or even cheese-covered nacho chips. On the No-Fail Diet, you may indulge in a treat once per week. (You'll notice that I say "one treat," not an entire day of overindulging.) Make this weekly treat part of your plan and do not feel guilty for enjoying it.

Keep your splurge to one treat per week, rather than planning to have smaller treats a few times per week. If you start adding in small indulgences, you'll get into the habit of wanting treats more often. Eventually those small treats will accumulate and be reflected by your bathroom scale. The occasional indulgence will not hinder your ability to lose weight. Instead, it will help you stick with your meal plan because you won't feel deprived. Remember that any changes you make to lose weight must be sustainable over the long term. Can you really see yourself giving up desserts, or chocolate, forever?

A Menu Plan for Phase 2 of the No-Fail Diet

Most of my clients want me to translate their meal plan into a menu of meals and snacks they can eat each day. Having a weekly menu plan makes it easy for them to shop for healthy foods and prepare their meals without any guesswork. Following a menu also helps my clients incorporate new foods and recipes into their eating plan—foods that they might not have tried before. You'll find a six-week menu of meal ideas and recipes in Chapter 6, The No-Fail Diet Menu Plans.

Phase 3: Maintaining Your Weight Loss

By the time you reach Phase 3, you have successfully completed 12 weeks on the No-Fail Diet. Congratulations! You have either achieved your weight-loss goal, or you are very close to doing so. If you still have more weight that you'd like to lose, continue following your Phase 2 meal plan until you reach your goal. The most common question clients ask me is, "How different will my diet be when I reach my weight goal?" My answer is always the same: Not much. The fact is, everything you do to lose weight must be the same things you do to keep that weight off. I remind clients that they can't go back to eating like they did when they were 20 pounds heavier, unless they want to weigh an extra 20 pounds.

Once you reach your weight goal, how much food you need to eat to maintain your weight will depend to a large extent on how physically active you are. If you ramp up the exercise, you can boost your calorie intake. If you stop exercising for a period of time, you need to cut back a little.

That's not to say you won't need to make adjustments to your diet once you reach your goal. As you approach your weight goal, two things may happen. What happens most often is that your rate of weight loss will slow down as you get close to your goal. Don't get discouraged; this is absolutely normal. It happens because your body is adapting to a lower calorie intake. As your body gets smaller in size, it requires fewer calories to perform the tasks than it did when you were heavier. Once you reach your goal weight, your calorie intake may have to be adjusted only slightly. The other thing that may occur is that once you reach your weight goal, you will continue to lose weight. To stop losing weight, you will definitely need to increase your calorie intake.

Determining how many calories you need to maintain your new weight is a process of trial and error. You can opt for a higher calorie level of the No-Fail Diet meal plan, or you can experiment by adding food to your diet in 100 calorie increments. Each week, add 100 calories to your daily diet and continue to monitor your weight. If you find your weight increases, you need to reduce your calorie intake— or add more exercise. When adding 100 calories worth of food to your diet, make sure you choose foods from the No-Fail Diet food groups. If adding foods such as crackers, rice cakes, or breakfast cereal, read the Nutrition Facts box to determine the serving size for 100 calories.

Start by adding foods that you miss in your diet, be it an extra fruit at breakfast, a glass of milk or soy milk with lunch, low-fat cheese in your sandwich, a larger portion size of rice at dinner, or a yogurt snack in the evening. The following table shows you the portion size for 100 calories worth of selected foods.

How Much Food Is 100 Calories*?

Protein Foods	Portion Size
Chicken	2 oz (60 g)
Lean meat	2 oz (60 g)
Halibut	2 1/2 oz (75 g)
Tuna	3 oz (90 g)
Salmon	2 oz (60 g)
Sole	2 1/2 oz (75 g)
Eggs	1 large
Cheese, part-skim	1 oz (30 g)
Cottage cheese, 1% MF**	1/2 cup (125 ml)
Chickpeas, cooked	1/3 cup (75 ml)
Kidney beans, cooked	1/2 cup (125 ml)
Lentils, cooked	1/2 cup (125 ml)

Milk and Milk Alternatives

Milk, skim or 1% MF	1 cup (250 ml)
Soy milk, plain, enriched	1 cup (250 ml)
Yogurt, 1% MF	1 cup (250 ml)

Starchy Foods

Bread, whole-grain	1 slice
Cereal (e.g., Bran Flakes, Cheerios)	1 cup (250 ml)
Cereal, 100% bran	1/2 cup (125 ml)
Oatmeal, cooked	3/4 cup (175 ml)
Pasta, cooked	1/2 cup (125 ml)
Popcorn, air popped	3 cups (750 ml)
Rice, cooked	1/2 cup (125 ml)

Fruits

Apple	1 medium
Applesauce	1 cup (250 ml)
Apricots	3
Banana	1 medium
Blueberries	1 cup (250 ml)
Dates	5
Fruit juice, unsweetened	3/4 to 1 cup (175 to 250 ml)
Orange	1 large
Pear	1 medium
Prunes	5
Raisins	1/4 cup (50 ml)
Strawberries	1 cup (250 ml)

Fats and Oils

Almonds, unsalted	14
Avocado	1/4
Cashews, unsalted	11
Peanut butter	1 tbsp (15 ml)
Peanuts, unsalted	17 (2 tbsp/25 ml)
Pecans	10 halves
Sunflower seeds	2 tbsp (25 ml)
Vegetable oil	2 tsp (10 ml)

* Calorie values range from 90 to 115.

** milk fat

You'll notice that I omitted the Vegetables food group from the list above. That's because I continue to encourage you to eat as many of these naturally low-calorie foods as you like. You should be eating at least 4 servings of colourful vegetables each day (1 serving is 1/2 cup/125 ml cooked or raw vegetables or 1 cup/250 ml mixed greens).

As you experiment with increasing your calorie intake, remember to always adhere to the four factors of the No-Fail Diet:

- *Timing.* Continue to eat every 3 to 4 hours to keep your blood sugar level stable and prevent hunger. Plan your meals and snacks times according to your daily schedule.

- *Protein.* Continue to have a high-protein food at every meal and in most snacks.

- *Portion size.* Continue to eyeball your portion sizes at meals so they don't creep up. Every so often, measure your foods to make sure you're not eating more than you think you are.

- *Tracking.* Continue to monitor your weight each week so that you are able to keep on top of small weight gains. Continue to keep tabs of your food intake with your Daily Food and Activity Tracker. This exercise will keep you aware of your food intake and help ensure your eating habits don't slip. When maintaining your weight, you may choose to continue to keep a food journal each day, or you may choose to track your food intake for 1 week each month. Assess your food journal regularly to identify areas that need improvement.

10 Strategies to Maintain Your Weight Loss

In Chapter 1, I asked you to determine your buffer zone, a 3 to 5 pound (1.5 to 2.5 kg) weight range that you will always maintain. Being successful at long-term weight control means that from this day forward, you will do what it takes to keep your weight within this range. Your buffer zone allows for a few extra pounds to accumulate from a vacation or string of social events. When your weight has crept to the upper number of your buffer zone, it's time to pull in the reins and get back on track. Once you return to your usual eating plan, your weight will settle at the lower end or middle of your buffer zone.

It takes work to maintain your weight. Keeping your weight stable requires the same level of commitment you made when deciding to lose weight. After all the hard work you've done to accomplish your goal, now is not the time to get sloppy. You need to stay on top of your food intake, your activity level, and all of the behaviours that helped you achieve your goal. The following 10 strategies will help you maintain your weight over the years to come. (As you'll notice, they are the same strategies you used to lose weight.)

1. *Plan ahead.* Not being organized is a surefire way to sabotage your healthy eating plan. If you come home from work, tired and hungry, to an empty fridge, chances are you'll order in, or graze your way through the evening. To eat healthfully during a hectic work week, plan your meals and snacks in advance, make time for grocery shopping, and batch cook on the weekend.

2. *Always eat breakfast.* Breakfast is a key ingredient in maintaining weight loss. The U.S.-based National Weight Control Registry, an ongoing study tracking the eating habits of over 5000 people who have successfully lost weight and kept it off, reported that 78% of participants eat breakfast every day of the week. Eating breakfast helps kick-start your metabolism and prevents you from getting too hungry before lunch. People who eat breakfast on a regular basis are more likely to have a structured eating plan throughout the day and are less likely to snack on empty calorie foods.

3. *Stick with your snacks.* The no-snacking approach can leave you feeling hungrier at meals and more likely to overeat. I can't emphasize enough how important it is to eat every 3 to 4 hours to help keep your blood sugar stable, your appetite under control, and your portion sizes down. Continue to eat the snacks you did while losing weight on the No-Fail Diet.

4. *Keep high-fat foods out of the house.* That's what 85% of weight-loss registrants say they do to help them stick with their weight maintenance diet. To stay on track, almost all say they stock their kitchen with plenty of healthy foods, and about one-third say they eat in restaurants less often.

5. *Be aware of extra nibbles.* It is easy to turn a blind eye to that piece of cheese you popped in your mouth when making the kids' lunches, or the repeated tastings when cooking dinner. But the scale keeps track of every calorie. Those mindless bites and sips can add up significantly—to an entire meal if you're not careful. Use your Food and Activity Tracker to identify mindless nibbling and plan strategies to prevent it. If you sample while you cook, chew sugarless gum, or sip on a glass of vegetable juice. If leftovers tempt you, cook only the amount you plan to serve.

6. *Don't deprive yourself.* People in the National Weight Control Registry say they don't give up their favourite foods. They continue to enjoy them, but not as often as they did when they were overweight. Continue to plan for your weekly indulgence on the weight maintenance phase.

7. *Don't let loose on the weekend.* A key to successful weight maintenance is consistency. Among my clients, the most successful are those who stick to their plans during the week and on the weekend. Research shows that people who don't give themselves a day or two off to cheat are one and a half times more likely to keep unwanted pounds off. Once you start giving yourself a few breaks on the weekend, you're more likely to ease off on Friday, and then Thursday. Eventually the breaks accumulate and show up on the bathroom scale. Although the times you eat may be different on the weekend, try to stick to your plan, and the No-Fail Diet principles, as closely as you can.

8. *Keep exercising.* If you want to prevent regaining your weight, exercise is essential. The majority of participants in the National Weight Control Registry (91%) say they exercise regularly to maintain their weight loss. Most combine walking with another type of planned exercise, such as aerobics classes, biking, or swimming. Regular exercise helps you stay trim by burning calories and increasing your metabolism. It also increases your motivation to eat a more healthful diet.

9. *Step on the scale regularly.* Weighing-in once a week gives you feedback on how well you are maintaining your weight. Data from the National Weight Control Registry indicates that frequent

weight monitoring is a critical factor in maintaining a weight loss. Among the 5000 participants studied, 75% say they weigh themselves at least once per week. Frequent weighing provides an early warning system. It allows you to catch small increases in weight quickly and take corrective action to prevent further weight gain. I recommend that you avoid weighing yourself every day, since normal daily fluctuations, mostly because of water weight, can be discouraging.

10. *Expect failure, but keep trying.* People who are successful at losing weight don't expect to be perfect. They consider lapses as momentary setbacks, not the ruin of all their hard work. Whether you've had a busy social schedule or you've just returned from a food-laden vacation, you're bound to put on a few pounds. As I mentioned above, the key to long-term weight maintenance is dealing with small weight gains when they occur. By telling yourself that you're human and it's okay to have slipped a little, you'll be amazed at how easy it is to return to your usual healthy routine.

5

The No-Fail 12-Week Fitness Program

Weight loss might be your number one reason for starting an exercise program, but I also want you to increase your overall fitness level. That's why the No-Fail 12-Week Fitness Program includes cardiovascular, strength, and flexibility exercises. The cardio component will help your body burn calories for weight loss and get your heart and lungs in shape. The strength-training exercises will help preserve your muscle mass and boost your metabolism. And finally, the flexibility exercises will help prevent muscle soreness and reduce the likelihood that you'll get injured during exercise.

The No-Fail 12-Week Fitness Program is designed for people who are new to exercise, for those who haven't worked out in some time, and for others who work out inconsistently (e.g., you get to the gym at most twice per week). You'll start slowly. Then gradually, each week, you'll be instructed to increase the amount of work your muscles perform so that further improvements can be made. When it comes to strength training, that means you'll increase the amount of weight you lift, or the number of sets or how many push-ups and sit-ups you do. To continue making fitness gains with cardiovascular exercise, you'll increase the speed of your walking, or add in a few hills, or notch up the resistance on the cardio machine at the gym. If you never change the intensity of the exercise you do, you'll hit a plateau, because your body adjusts to anything you do repeatedly.

If you're already an exercise buff, keep up the good work. But if you're cruising through your workout, it's time to pick up the pace and challenge yourself by increasing the intensity or adding in new exercises. If you always climb on the same old machine and press the same buttons, you might very well be undermining your results. In Chapter 2, I gave you tips to help you stay motivated and stick to your workout routine. The No-Fail 12-Week Fitness Tracker in Appendix 1 will help you monitor the results of your fitness program.

Before You Start Exercising

Most healthy people can safely start an exercise program. However, if you're a man over 45 or a woman over 55 and have not been regularly active, or you have any health concerns, consult your doctor first. Regardless of your age, consult with your doctor if you have two or more of the following risk factors:

* High blood pressure
* High blood cholesterol
* Diabetes
* You're a smoker.
* You have a family history of early onset heart disease (father before the age of 55 or mother before the age of 65).

Other reasons to visit your doctor before starting an exercise program include:

* You feel pain in your chest during physical activity.
* In the past you have felt pain in your chest when you were not active.
* You sometimes lose your balance or become dizzy.
* You have a bone or joint condition that could be made worse by exercise.

Your Preparation Checklist

Before you hit the pavement, the gym, or your basement, it's important to have the proper exercise equipment, to prevent injuries. On the No-Fail 12-Week Fitness Program, you'll need the following:

Proper shoes. You might not need to buy a new pair of shoes, but you must make sure that those that you have are in good shape. If you're exercising in the same pair of running shoes that you used in high school gym class or that you have walked in for the past few years, they need replacing. If you notice your knees and ankles get sore when working out, your shoes could be the culprit. Find a sporting goods store that has a qualified salesperson who can help fit the right pair of shoes for you.

Water bottle. You should always have water while you're working out, especially when exercising in hot, humid weather. When you exercise, your muscles generate heat. This heat must be released from your body as sweat or else your performance will be impaired. If you lose too much sweat during exercise and become dehydrated, the fluid in your bloodstream can't circulate efficiently to your working muscles and your skin. As a result, you'll produce less sweat, causing your muscles to build up heat. Dehydration is one of the most common causes of early fatigue during exercise.

To prevent dehydration, drink at least 2 cups (500 ml) of water up to 2 hours before you begin your workout. Invest in a good water bottle that you can use at the gym, or strap to your waist when exercising outside. Drink water at a rate of 1/2 to 1 cup (125 to 250 ml) every 15 to 20 minutes during exercise. Once you've finished your workout, drink at least 2 cups (500 ml) of water to replace the fluids that you've lost from sweating.

Dumbbells. If you will be working out in your home, you will need pairs of dumbbells, also known as free weights, of varying weight. If you want to have all your bases covered, and have room to increase your strength, purchase pairs of dumbbells in weights of 3, 5, 8, 10, 12, and 15 pounds (or 1.5, 2, 2.5, 5, and 7 kg). However, if you are new to strength training, all you really need to start are 3, 5, 8, and 10 pound (1.5, 2, 2.5, and 5 kg) dumbbells. You can always buy heavier weights as your strength increases. You'll also need to purchase an exercise mat.

Following the No-Fail Diet 12-Week Fitness Program, you should be feeling fatigue in the last 3 or 4 repetitions of those exercises that involve dumbbells. If you are not, you need to move up to a heavier weight.

Resistance bands.   These exercise bands are essentially giant rubber bands with plastic handles that you pull against to strengthen certain muscle groups. Resistance bands come in a range of resistance levels, from easy to stretch, to progressively more difficult. If you're a beginning strength trainer, start at the lowest level of resistance and work your way to higher levels. One typical way of using the resistance band is to place the end of the band under your feet while standing, hold the other end in one or both hands, and pull up against the band. This is the equivalent of a bicep curl with hand weights. Many of the strength exercises in the No-Fail 12-Week Fitness Program can be done with resistance bands instead of dumbbells. You'll find books on how to use exercise bands in the fitness section of your local bookstore.

Resistance bands are relatively inexpensive and easy to use. And they are great to have with you when you travel so that you can continue your strength training while you're away from home. You can pack them right inside your running shoe. Exercise bands must be kept out of direct sunlight so that they don't get brittle and dry and more likely to break. Before you start your strength workout, always inspect your band for any holes that may have been caused by your running shoes. A hole in your exercise band decreases its integrity and increases the chances that it will snap on you.

Exercise ball.   Also called a stability ball, this inflatable ball is used to strengthen muscles, improve posture, and help prevent back pain. You can do almost any strength exercise with an exercise ball—shoulder presses, bicep curls, sit-ups, even push-ups. Sitting and balancing on the ball while you're lifting weight requires you to engage your core muscles (all the muscles attached to your spine) to keep yourself upright on the ball.

When you purchase a ball, it is not inflated; check to see if it comes with a pump. Some brands require you to purchase a pump separately. Exercise balls come in five sizes. At the fitness equipment store, ask the salesperson to help you choose the right one for your height.

Clothing and sunblock. When you exercise, wear loose-fitting clothes that allow you to move freely and feel comfortable. In the summer, wearing light colours will help you keep cooler outdoors when the weather is warm. Dark clothes, which trap light, will help keep you warmer in the winter. Choose thick, cotton-blend exercise socks to prevent blisters and keep your feet dry.

You'll also need to wear clothing that has a wicking property. This means it pulls sweat away from your body to keep your skin dry, helping to keep you cool in summer and warm in winter. If you exercise outdoors in the evening near traffic (e.g., jogging or power walking), wear light-coloured clothing and reflective bands so drivers can see you. During the cooler winter months, you will need to wear three layers, starting with a thermal base layer that's tight fitting, wicking, and warm. Your middle layer should provide more insulation; its function is to pull the moisture from the base layer out to the outer layer. As the weather gets colder, you will want to add this layer, especially if you are going to be walking for a long period. The amount of insulation desired is also dependent on your personal preference: If you get hot quickly, you may want to stick with a lighter insulation layer. The mid-layer should be a bit looser than the base layer, but it still needs to maintain contact with the base layer. Common materials for a mid-layer are down, polyester, fleece, and synthetic materials. Many mid-layers may have added ventilation for when you warm up. Pit zips, long zippers, adjustable collars, and cuffs provide a way to moderate your body temperature throughout your workout.

Finally, wear an outer layer that will block the wind. Always use a sunblock to protect against sunburn and skin cancers, regardless of the season.

12 Weeks of Fitness with Trina Lambe

I help people lose weight every day in my private practice by developing customized nutrition plans for them and giving general exercise advice. But I don't design detailed fitness programs for my clients; I leave that for the fitness professionals. And that is precisely what I have done for this book: I enlisted my own fitness coach, Trina Lambe, to design the No-Fail 12-Week Fitness Program. I love working out with Trina—her enthusiasm for fitness is contagious and she doesn't let me slack off. With credentials like hers, I feel like a slouch if I don't push through my workouts.

Trina is a certified personal trainer, a spinning instructor, and a darn good figure skater (she skated competitively for 7 years). If that's not enough, she's also a seasoned mountain bike racer who competes in both the Ontario Cup and Canada Cup racing circuits. And there's more. In 2004 and 2005 she won first place in the Ottawa Carlton Cup Triathlon. She balances her high-energy sports with daily yoga.

Below I've outlined Trina's fitness program week by week (you'll see Trina in the accompanying photographs, demonstrating the exercises). Each week you will do four cardiovascular workouts of varying duration and intensities, three 30-minute strength-training workouts, and four 5-minute stretching sessions (you'll stretch after each cardio workout).

Cardio Workouts

The No-Fail 12-Week Fitness Program requires you to complete four cardio workouts each week. To get an optimum workout, you'll need to pace your cardio exercise. You want your heart rate at the proper intensity level for an extended period. If your heart rate gets too high, your activity can become counterproductive; if it is too low, you are not getting any substantial health benefits. During each cardio workout, you'll be asked to monitor your heart rate or perceived rate of exertion (PRE). For a review of PRE and heart rate calculations, see page 36 in Chapter 2.

Two Standard Cardio Workouts

For your Standard Cardio, you will start with 15 minutes of continuous exercise, working at a level 7 PRE or 70% of your maximum heart rate. If you have never exercised before, start at 50% of your maximum heart rate or level 5 PRE: Work up to level 7 RPE or 70% of your maximum heart rate, the level prescribed in the No-Fail 12-Week Fitness Program, and then start the program. For example, if when you start working at level 7 you can maintain that for only 7 minutes, work from that 7 minute–mark and increase it by 2 minutes per week until you can do the full 15 minutes at level 7 before beginning the program.

Each week, your Standard Cardio workouts will increase by 2 minutes in duration. By the end of the 12-week program, you'll be able to sustain your cardio workout for 37 minutes. If you are already comfortable doing a 30-minute workout, that's fantastic. I suggest you start your program with 30 minutes of Standard Cardio and increase your workouts by 2 minutes every 2 weeks. Within 3 months you'll be comfortable doing a 54-minute cardio workout.

You can choose to exercise on any piece of cardio equipment at the gym or to power walk or jog outside. I encourage you to try a number of different ways to do your cardio. One day you may power walk, the next use the elliptical trainer. Each piece of equipment works your muscles differently and gives you a different calorie burn. You may have days where your knees are bothering you, and in this case swimming or cycling may be a better option than going outside to pound the pavement.

We all have our favourite cardio machines. Try not to get stuck in the rut of always using the same piece of equipment. You need to step into that uncomfortable zone to get the results you want.

One Interval Cardio Workout

Interval training is an important part of your exercise program, as it helps strengthen your heart, condition your muscles, and burn calories. Your intervals are very short, 2 minutes at most. One complete interval consists of a work phase, followed by an active recovery phase.

In the No-Fail 12-Week Fitness Program, you will be asked to do only four intervals in each workout, but the work phase will increase in duration as the weeks progress.

During the work phase, I want you to give it your all. Work as hard as you can to spend the designated time at level 8 PRE or 80% of your maximum heart rate. While you are breathing hard and working those muscles, remind yourself that this is only for a minute or two. You want to work, work, work.

During the active recovery phase of the interval, you will get your heart rate down to level 6 PRE or 60% of your maximum heart rate. As you train your heart, this will become easier and easier. When you are starting out, it's okay if it takes you longer than a couple of minutes to get to level 6 PRE or 60% of your maximum heart rate. It's the getting there that is most important. As you become fitter, the time it takes your heart rate to slow down will decrease. Active recovery does not mean that you totally stop exercising—hence the word active. You need to still be working during this phase, just not at the same level of intensity as you were during the work phase of your interval.

Here are two tips to help you get your heart rate down during the active recovery phase of interval training:

- Take a quick scan of your body. If you're gripping anything, or if your shoulders are up at your ears, there is tension in your body. Let it go. You are wasting energy and preventing your heart rate from slowing.

- Keep in mind that you finished a phase of exercise that made you breathe vigorously. Slow your breath by controlling your breathing. Take deeper breaths, inhaling through your nose and exhaling through your mouth.

One Extended Cardio Workout

This workout is one and a half times longer than your Standard Cardio workout but at a slightly lower intensity. For example, if your Standard Cardio workout is 15 minutes, your once weekly Extended Cardio workout is 22 minutes. Each week, as you increase the duration of your

Standard Cardio workouts, you will also increase the duration of your Extended Cardio. To help pass the time during extended cardio, you may want to listen to your IPod or books-on-tape, or watch television. But don't forget about the task at hand. You need to be working at level 6 RPE or 60% of your maximum heart rate.

Using Cardio Equipment at the Gym

You'll find the following standard cardio equipment at the gym. Try each of them out to see what works best for you.

Treadmill

When you first step on the treadmill, familiarize yourself with all of the buttons. Know where the stop button is and how to use it. Most treadmills have a safety clip that you can attach to your clothing. The safety clip has a string that attaches to the machine. It allows you to stop the power if you're feeling unsafe, faint, ill, or hurt. Treadmills also have side rails, but these are not to be used while walking or running. Hanging on to the side rails does not simulate actual walking or running and can cause posture, body alignment, and balance problems. Holding on to the side rails results in a less effective workout—you'll burn up to 30% fewer calories.

Standard treadmills have two features: speed and incline. Start by stepping on the centre of the belt, then slowly increase your speed. Although it can vary from person to person, in general, a brisk walking pace is 3.8 to 4.0 miles (6.1 to 6.4 km) per hour. If you're tall, you might walk as fast as 4.5 miles (7.2 km) per hour. Find a pace on the treadmill that allows you to achieve your desired heart rate goals.

The incline on a treadmill simulates a hill. You can increase the grade of the belt in 0.5% increments, starting at a 0% grade (perfectly flat) all the way to a 15% grade (a steep hill). When you use the incline feature for the first time, you will likely want to grip the side rails, but avoid this temptation. If you have back or knee problems, stick with an incline of zero or 0.5%.

Many treadmills have a heart rate control. Those with a handgrip heart rate control require holding on to the sensors located on the side rails. This is awkward for walking, and just not possible for jogging. Some treadmills have a wireless control, which is much easier to use while you're moving your body. You attach a strap around your chest, and your heart rate is fed to the console.

As you improve your fitness on the 12-week program, you'll reach points when you need to speed up the pace in order to achieve your target heart rate goal. If you are not comfortable with jogging and prefer to walk, use the incline button to increase your exercise intensity. When you add an incline, your heart rate will increase as you walk up the hill.

The incline is a great feature to use for your interval workouts (you will be asked to do one each week). When you need to be in the work phase (level 8 or 80% of your maximum heart rate), increase the incline so that you are going up a hill. Your heart rate will increase. You'll notice that it doesn't take much of an incline to speed up your heart rate. When doing intervals, start with a 3% incline for the work phase. If you don't get your heart rate to 80%, increase the incline as needed.

During your interval workout you can use speed to increase your heart rate, rather than incline. Simply move from walking at 3.8 miles (6.1 km) per hour (active recovery phase) to running at 6.0 to 6.5 miles (9.7 to 10.5 km) per hour (work phase). Both methods are effective for interval training; you will need to decide which you are most comfortable with.

Elliptical Trainer

The elliptical trainer operates in the same fashion as a treadmill in terms of incline and resistance. When you use the incline (or ramp) on the elliptical trainer you will be using different muscles than when you are on the flat setting. As you climb, you use more butt and quad (front of thighs) muscles. For the incline, use level 6. This is a level that works two of the largest muscle groups in your body.

On the machine, you'll notice a "strides per minute" display. The number displayed is the speed you are moving at. During your Standard Cardio workout and your Extended Cardio workout, it is important to keep this number consistent at about 130 to 150 strides per minute. During your Interval Cardio workout, this number can increase to 225 strides per minute.

You will use the incline and resistance features to modify your heart rate. Resistance is the amount of friction the machine creates to slow down your strides per minute. That means that as the resistance increases, you need to work harder (and burn more calories) to maintain a constant number of strides per minute. Find a moderate resistance that keeps your heart rate in the target zone of 50% to 70% of your maximum heart rate. If there is no resistance on the machine (that is, the resistance level is zero), momentum will be propelling the movement instead of your muscles.

Stationary Bike

Stationary bikes offer you many choices. The upright bike is most like a pedal bicycle you would ride outdoors. There are also recumbent bikes, in which you sit back with your legs outstretched in front of you. Both bikes are great choices for non-weight-bearing cardiovascular exercise, a type of activity suited for anyone with knee or back problems. Which bike you prefer is ultimately a matter of which is most comfortable for you to ride. When you sit on the bike, the height of the seat is most important. You should have a slight bend in your knee when your leg is fully extended.

You can modify the speed of the bike by your own power. When looking at the display, you will see an RPM (revolutions per minute) number. During a bike workout, it's recommended that you consistently pedal at 80 to 90 RPM. Stationary bikes also have an incline/ hill component, called the resistance.

StairMaster

Working out on the StairMaster simulates walking up stairs, at a very low impact. This upright machine has handrails to use for balance, but they're not intended to rest on while you are working out. If you do, you're not working as hard as you should be, and your calorie burn will be less. The StairMaster has two variables that influence how many calories you burn: resistance and step rate (steps climbed per minute). The resistance is determined by which level (1 to 20) you select on the display monitor. The higher the level, the more resistance the machine creates for you to work against. In other words, the higher the level, the harder you have to work and the more calories you will burn.

If you've never used the StairMaster before, start at a resistance of level 3. You need to step fast enough so that the steps, or pedals, don't touch the floor or top of the machine. Your body should be upright while you are stair climbing. If you find you need to use the handrails to hold on or lean on the control panel, you need to lower the resistance. Most StairMasters have a heart rate control, which allows you to monitor your workout intensity. If your heart rate is below your target, you need to increase the resistance. If it's too high, work out at a level lower.

All types of cardio equipment have set programs—Quick Start, Manual, Fitness Test, Fat Burner, Calorie Burner, Speed Intervals, and Heart Rate Zone Trainer, and so on. For the No-Fail 12-Week Fitness Program, use the quick start button, or manual program, and enter the length of time you plan to work out on the equipment. Your weekly interval workouts give specific directions as to how long you must stay in the work and active recovery phases and what your target heart rate should be. The interval programs on machines will not be the same as what is prescribed for you in Trina's No Fail 12-Week Fitness Program.

Strength Exercises

On the No-Fail 12-Week Fitness Program, you will do a 30-minute strength-training workout 3 days per week. During each strength workout you will work your upper body, your lower body, and your core. Your body's core—the area around your trunk and pelvis—is where your centre of gravity is located. Think of your core as the foundation of your body; it's the area that supports your spine for just about any activity. Strengthening your core muscles will improve your posture and help reduce back pain and injury.

If you are not doing your strength workout after your cardio workout, warm up with 5 minutes of light aerobic activity to get your circulation going and your joints moving. Always breathe regularly when doing your strength exercises. To allow your muscles to rest, take a day off between strength-training sessions.

Breaking Up Your Strength Workouts

If you're pressed for time, you can break up your strength-training workouts to make them more manageable. If you prefer, you can do the upper body and core exercises in the morning and the lower body exercises in the evening. Or you can do your three types of strength exercises (upper, lower, core) at three different times during the day. Do whatever works best for your schedule. You might even carry your resistance band in your purse and use it for 10 minutes on your lunch break.

When breaking up your strength workout into smaller sections, do not split up sets. The designated number of sets and repetitions help build muscle strength and endurance. Doing one set first and another one hours later defeats the purpose of the number of sets and repetitions intended for each exercise. Also, keep like sections together: upper body, lower body, and core exercise.

As your strength increases each week, the intensity of your workouts will change so that you can continue making fitness improvements. Every 3 weeks you will be given a new series of strength exercises, to keep you interested. The strength exercises that you will find in the No-Fail 12-Week Fitness Program are outlined below.

Weeks 1, 2, and 3: Upper Body

Bicep Curl

Target Area
Front upper arms (biceps)

Equipment needed
Dumbbells

Set-up
Stand tall in your upper body, your feet shoulder width apart and your knees slightly bent. Keep your toes pointed forward. Hold a dumbbell in each hand, palms facing forward.

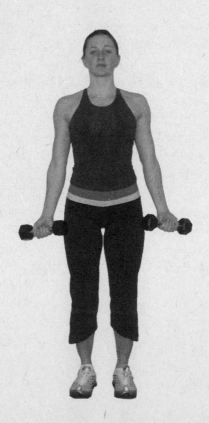

Movement

Contract your abdominal muscles and, bending your elbows, bring your hands with the dumbbells up to your shoulders. Your palms should face your shoulders. Pause, then slowly lower your hands to starting position. Control your movement throughout each repetition: Only your arms should be working, not any other part of your body. Exhale as you lift your arms, and inhale as you lower to starting position. Repeat for 12 repetitions to complete one set.

Tip

You should be feeling fatigue in the front of your arms on the last 3 or 4 repetitions. If you are not, you need to move up to a heavier weight. This rule applies to every exercise that you do with dumbbells.

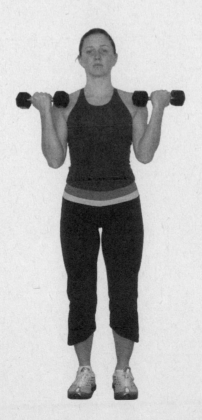

Overhead Triceps

Target area
Back upper arms (triceps)

Equipment needed
Dumbbell

Set-up
Stand with your feet slightly apart and your knees slightly bent, your arms fully extended above your head. Hold one dumbbell with both hands, in an interlocking grip.

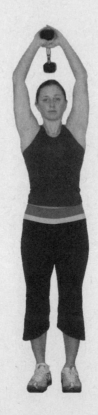

Movement

Contract your abdominal muscles and slowly lower the dumbbell behind your head until your forearms are parallel to the floor. Pause, then gradually raise the dumbbell to starting position. Control your movement throughout the exercise, keeping the movement slow. Inhale as you bring your forearms parallel to the floor, behind your head, and exhale as you stretch up your arms overhead. Repeat for 12 repetitions to complete one set.

Tip

Keep your arms close to your head and maintain your posture so that you do not arch your back.

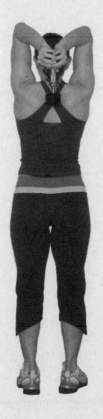

Lat Pull Down

Target area
Upper back (latissimus dorsi, biceps)

Equipment needed
Dumbbells, chair, or exercise ball

Set-up
Sit upright on the chair or exercise ball with your feet flat on the floor, your back straight, and your hips and shoulders aligned. Hold one dumbbell in each hand. Bring your arms up over your head, your palms facing forward and the dumbbells touching end to end.

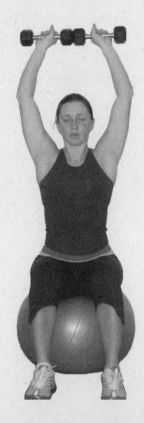

Movement

Contract your abdominal muscles and slowly bend your elbows, lowering your hands so that your upper arms are parallel to the floor and your elbows are bent at 90 degrees. Think of your elbows leading as you start this movement. Pause at the bottom of the movement. Exhale as you lower your arms, and inhale as you raise your arms to starting position. Continue to keep your abdominals squeezed tight to support your back, being careful not to arch. Repeat for 12 repetitions to complete one set.

Tip

At the bottom of the movement, look across to your elbows to make sure they are aligned with your shoulders and that your upper arms are parallel to the floor, straight out from your shoulders. Do not let your upper arms drop below your shoulders.

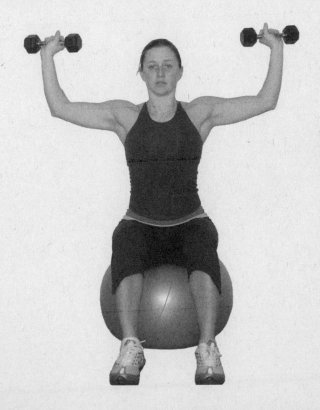

Chest Fly

Target area
Chest (pectorals major, pectorals minor)

Equipment needed
Dumbbells, exercise mat

Set-up
Lie on your back on the mat with your knees bent and your feet flat on the floor. Extend your arms straight over your chest, over the midline of your body, palms facing inward so that the dumbbells are touching.

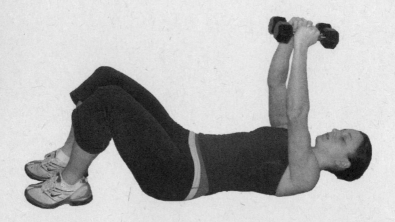

Movement

Contract your abdominal muscles and slowly lower your arms to the floor, palms still facing inward. Keep your arms straight but not hyperextended. Lower the dumbbells until your upper arms just touch the floor. Pause, then slowly raise your arms back to starting position. Inhale as your arms move out wide, and exhale as you bring them back to your starting position. Both arms are working at the same time and moving fluidly. Repeat for 12 repetitions to complete one set.

Tip

Keep your head and neck on the floor and relaxed. To increase difficulty and further engage your abdominal muscles, take your feet off the floor and place them in a tabletop-like position so your shins are parallel to the ceiling.

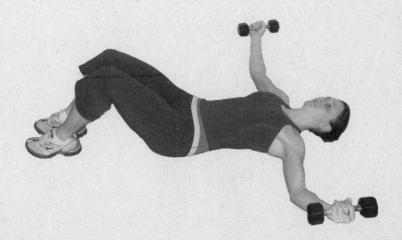

Weeks 1, 2, and 3: Lower Body

Basic Squat

Target area
Upper legs (quadriceps and hamstrings)

Equipment needed
None

Set-up
Stand tall in your upper body, your feet slightly wider than shoulder width apart. Keep your toes pointed forward, your arms resting at your sides.

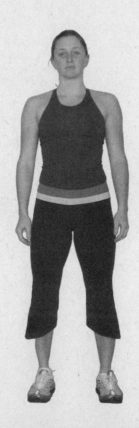

Movement

Contract your abdominal muscles. Keeping your upper body strong, bend your knees, gradually lowering yourself until your thighs are almost parallel to the floor. Keep your weight back, on your heels. Pause at the bottom of the squat and then slowly rise up. Inhale as you bend, and exhale as you return to starting position. Control your movement throughout the exercise. Your upper body will lean slightly forward; this is okay as long as your shoulders do not go past your knees. Your back remains straight. Repeat for 12 repetitions to complete one set.

Tip

As you do this exercise, check that your knees are moving overtop your toes, and not to the inside or outside of your feet. The bend in your knees should not exceed 90 degrees.

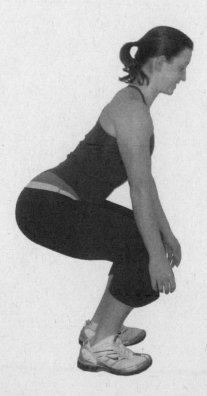

Static Forward Lunge

Target area
Legs (quadriceps, hamstrings, calves)

Equipment needed
None

Set-up
Stand with your feet slightly wider than hip width apart, one foot in front of the other. Stretch your back leg behind you so that the heel is off the floor and the knee is extended. Bend your front leg, making sure your knee does not extend beyond the toes. Rest your arms at your sides. Your shoulders should be directly over your hips.

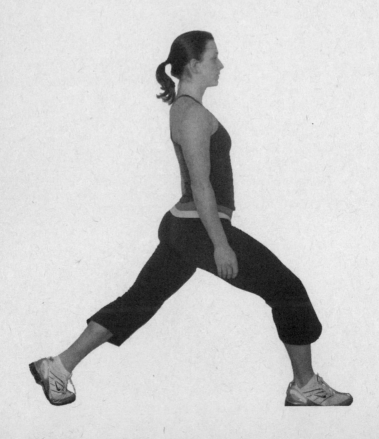

Movement

Contract your abdominal muscles and slowly bend your back knee. As your lunge deepens, your front knee will also bend deeper, but still do not let it extend past the toes. Lower yourself until you feel a stretch in the leg that is behind. Pause, then slowly rise to starting position. Exhale as you bend, and inhale as you rise. Repeat for 12 repetitions, then switch legs and repeat for another 12 to complete one set.

Tip

If you are getting your back leg down to the floor without feeling a stretch in the front of that thigh, reach that leg back farther so that you get a stretch when you are halfway to the floor.

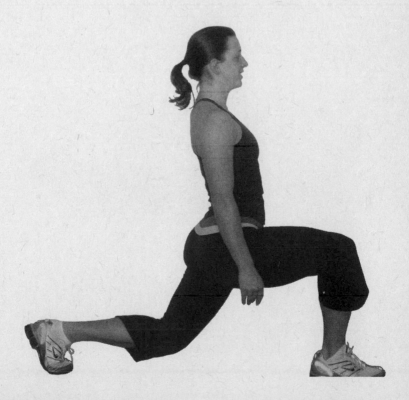

Lying Leg Curl

Target area

Back upper legs (hamstrings)

Equipment needed

Exercise mat

Set-up

Lie face down on the mat and bring your hands beneath you, slightly wider than shoulder width apart, palms down. With your gaze directed to the floor, squeeze your legs together, then bend one leg slightly so that the foreleg is 1 inch (2.5 cm) off the floor. This is the leg that will do the movement.

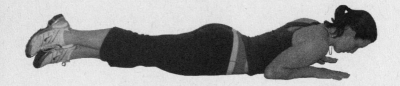

Movement
Contract your abdominal muscles. With the leg that is off the floor, slowly move your heel closer to your bum. This action is done to a count of four. Pause, then lower your leg to starting position. Exhale as you squeeze toward your bum, and inhale as you return to starting position. Repeat for 12 repetitions, then switch legs and repeat for another 12 to complete one set.

Tip
Keep your thighs and your buttocks squeezing together throughout the exercise.

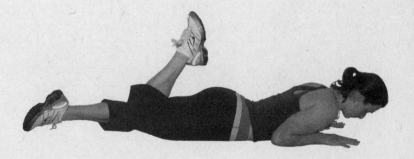

Calf Raise, Both Feet

Target area

Lower legs (gastrocnemius, soleus)

Equipment needed

Rolled-up bath towel or bottom step of a staircase

Set-up

Stand tall in your upper body, your feet slightly wider than shoulder width apart. Keep your toes pointed forward and the balls of your feet on the towel roll or step.

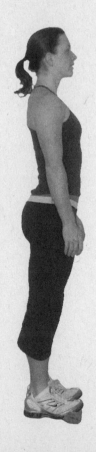

Movement

Contract your abdominal muscles and slowly lift your body upward so that you are standing tip-toe. Hold for a moment, then slowly lower. Keep your back straight and your arms at your sides. Exhale as you lift, and inhale as you lower. Repeat for 12 repetitions to complete one set.

Tip

Keep your feet straight so that you don't twist your ankle. Think about balance.

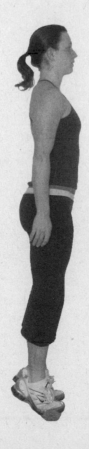

Weeks 1, 2, and 3: Core Exercises

Basic Crunch

Target area
Abdominals (rectus abdominis)

Equipment needed
Exercise mat

Set-up
Lie on your back on the mat with your knees bent and your feet flat on the floor. Clasp your hands lightly behind your head, your elbows wide to the sides.

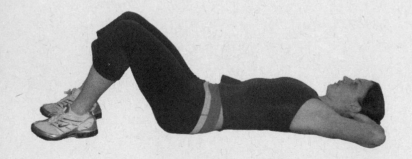

Movement

Contract your abdominal muscles to power you forward, and slowly lift your head, neck, and shoulders off the mat. Your chin should be pointed forward, not tucked into your chest. Pause, then slowly lower. Exhale as you lift, and inhale as you return to starting position. Repeat for 12 repetitions to complete one set.

Tip

Don't let your neck roll when you are lifting up: Keep it straight. Focus on a spot on the ceiling and lift your head, neck, shoulders, and chest up to it. Keep your chin off your chest (imagine you're holding an orange between your chin and your chest; maintain this distance).

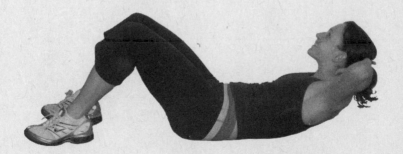

Side Bridge

Target area

Sides of torso (quadratus lumborum, abdominal obliques)

Equipment needed

Exercise mat

Set-up

Lie on your side on the mat with your shoulders, hips, and legs aligned. Bend your legs to create a right angle at your knee. Place your top arm on your hip. Place the elbow of your bottom arm under the shoulder. The forearm of your bottom arm should be on the floor and the upper part of this arm should be supporting the shoulder.

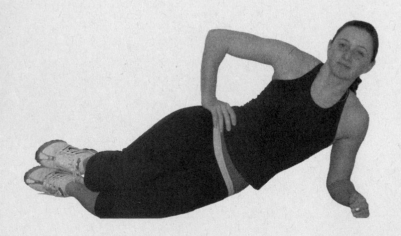

Movement

Contract your abdominal muscles and lift your hip off the mat. Your knees and bottom elbow should be on the floor supporting you. Hold for 10 to 15 seconds. If you find holding for 15 seconds easy, increase the time gradually. Keep your inhalation and exhalation fluid and rhythmical with deep breaths. Repeat on the other side to complete one set.

Tip

Keep looking forward. The tendency is for your hips to twist; avoid doing so by engaging your abdominal muscles for support.

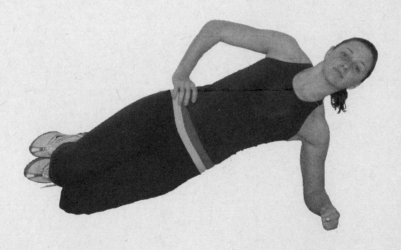

Wall Push-Up

Target area

Shoulders and torso

Equipment needed

Wall

Set-up

Stand on the floor facing a wall. You should be approximately 2 to 3 feet (0.5 to 1.0 m) from the wall. Extend your arms in front of you, lean forward, and place your hands on the wall, slightly wider than shoulder width apart (although you can place your hands closer or wider if you prefer). At this point, your arms should be straight and

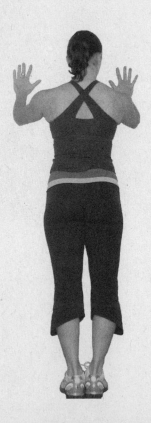

parallel to the floor, and your feet should be flat on the floor. Check that your body forms a straight line from shoulders to ankles. This is the starting position.

Movement

Contract your abdominal muscles. Bend your elbows and lower your body toward the wall until your face is nearly touching. Straighten your arms, pressing your body away from the wall. Inhale as you lower your body toward the wall, and exhale as you return to starting position. Your body should remain in a straight position throughout the exercise. Repeat for 12 repetitions to complete one set.

Tip

Keep your heels on the floor.

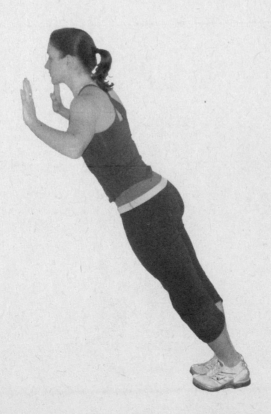

Weeks 4, 5, and 6: Upper Body

Hammer Curl

Target area

Front upper arms (biceps)

Equipment needed

Dumbbells

Set-up

Stand tall in your upper body, your feet shoulder width apart and your knees slightly bent. Keep your toes pointed forward. Hold one dumbbell in each hand, arms at your sides, palms facing inward.

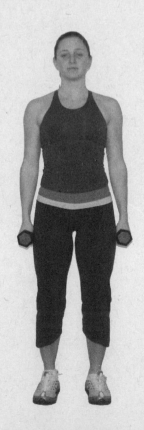

Movement

Contract your abdominal muscles. Slowly raise one arm so that the dumbbell meets your shoulder. Keep your palm facing inward. Pause, then slowly lower your arm to starting position. Control your movement throughout the exercise: You want only your arms to do the movement, not any other part of your body. Exhale as you lift, and inhale as you lower. Repeat for 12 repetitions, then switch arms and repeat for another 12 to complete one set.

Tip

Keep your palms facing inward to emulate the movement of hammering a nail. Don't let your body sway: Be steady.

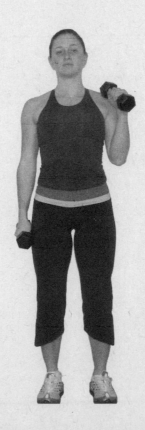

Triceps Kickback

Target area
Back upper arms (triceps)

Equipment needed
Dumbbells

Set-up
Stand with your feet slightly apart and your knees slightly bent, your upper body bent forward so that your back is parallel to the floor. With one dumbbell in each hand, bend your elbows and bring your arms up to brush your sides so that your elbow is higher than your back and your arms are close to your sides. Your arms should be bent at 90 degrees.

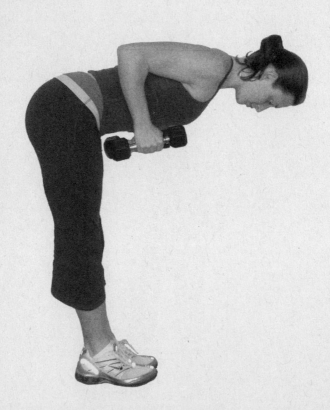

Movement

Contract your abdominal muscles and slowly extend your arms straight out behind you, hinging at your elbow joints, palms facing inward. Pause when your arms are extended, then slowly bring them back to starting position. Exhale on the arm stretch backwards, and inhale as your arms return to starting position. Control your movement throughout the exercise—no swaying. Keep your torso strong and flat. Repeat for 12 repetitions to complete one set.

Tip

Keep your arms close to your body and palms facing inward. You should not be moving your shoulders; the only movement comes from bending your elbows.

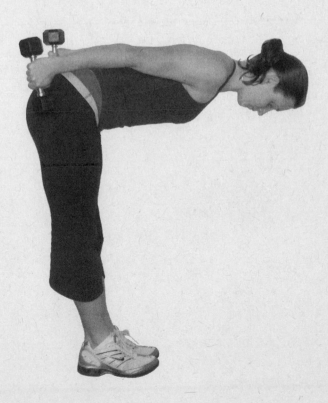

Chest Press

Target area
Chest and upper back (pectoralis major, pectoralis minor, triceps)

Equipment needed
Dumbbells, bench or exercise mat

Set-up
Lie on your back on a bench or on a mat if you do not have a bench. With your knees bent and feet flat on the floor, press your lower back into the bench so that it is not arched. Extend your arms straight over your chest, holding the dumbbells end to end, your palms facing inward.

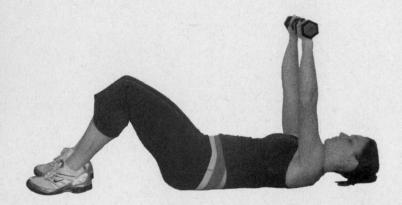

Movement

Contract your abdominal muscles and slowly bend your elbows until your upper arm almost touches the floor if using a mat, or are parallel to the floor if using a bench. Pause, then slowly raise your arms back to starting position. Inhale as you lower the dumbbells toward the floor, and exhale as you raise them to starting position. Control the movement and keep your lower back pressing into the bench or mat. Repeat for 12 repetitions to complete one set.

Tip

Be sure to contract your abdominal muscles so that there is no arch in your back.

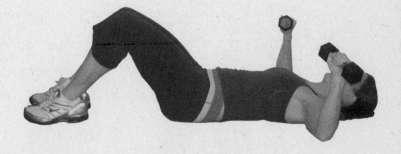

Standing Forward Row

Target area

Shoulders (deltoids)

Equipment needed

Dumbbells

Set-up

Stand tall in your upper body, your feet slightly wider than shoulder width apart and your arms straight. Hold one dumbbell in each hand with your palms resting against your thighs and facing inward.

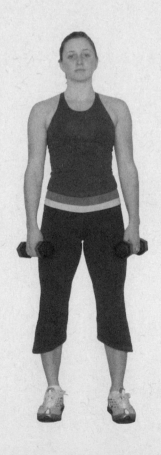

Movement

Contract your abdominal muscles. With your elbows pointed outward, slowly pull the dumbbells up in front of you, brushing your body. Lead with your elbows, stopping at shoulder height. Pause, then slowly lower to starting position. Exhale as you lift, and inhale as you lower. Repeat for 12 repetitions to complete one set.

Tip

You don't need to lift your elbows higher than your shoulders. Your palms should always be facing inward.

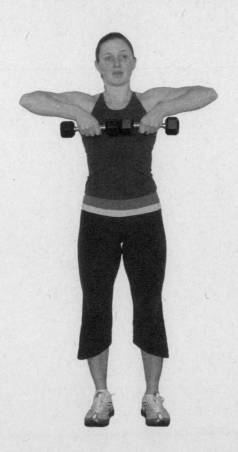

Weeks 4, 5, and 6: Lower Body

Basic Squat with Weights

Target area
Upper legs (quadriceps and hamstrings)

Equipment needed
Dumbbells

Set-up
Stand tall in your upper body, your feet slightly wider than shoulder width apart. Keep your toes pointed forward. Hold one dumbbell in each hand, your arms resting at your sides.

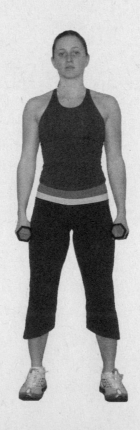

Movement

Contract your abdominal muscles. Keeping your upper body strong, bend your knees, gradually lowering your body until your thighs are almost parallel to the floor. Keep your body weight back, on your heels, and your arms resting at your sides. Pause, then slowly rise. Inhale as you lower, and exhale as you rise. Control your movement throughout the exercise. Your upper body will lean slightly forward; this is okay as long as it is only slightly. Repeat for 12 repetitions to complete one set.

Tip

Keep a loose grip on the dumbbells (don't clench them) and your shoulders down, away from your ears. If your shoulders are past your knees, you are too far forward.

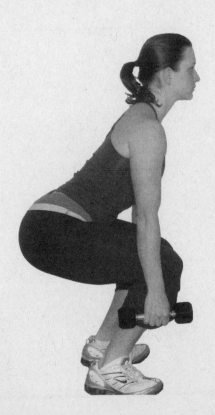

Static Forward Lunge with Weights

Target area
Legs (quadriceps, hamstrings, calves)

Equipment needed
Dumbbells

Set-up
Stand with your feet slightly wider than hip width apart, one leg stretched out in front of the other with the knee slightly bent. Make sure the knee is not extended past the toes. Stretch your back leg so that the heel is off the floor. Rest your arms at your sides, one dumbbell in each hand. You should be able to draw a straight line from your shoulders to your hips.

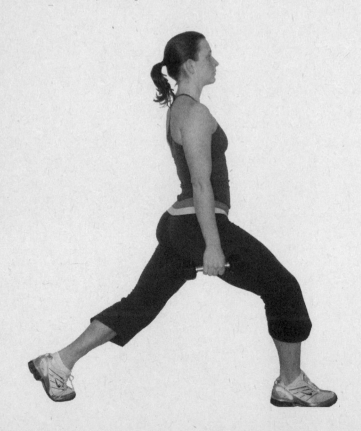

Movement

Contract your abdominal muscles. Slowly bend your back knee. As your lunge deepens, your front knee should bend deeper, but it still should not extend past the toes. Lower yourself until you feel a stretch in the leg that is behind. Continue to rest your arms at your sides, dumbbells in hands. Pause, then slowly rise to starting position. Exhale as you lower, and inhale as you return to starting position. Repeat for 12 repetitions, then switch legs and repeat for another 12 to complete one set.

Tip

If you don't feel a stretch in the front of your thigh of the leg that is behind, reach that leg back farther so that you feel a stretch when you are halfway to the floor.

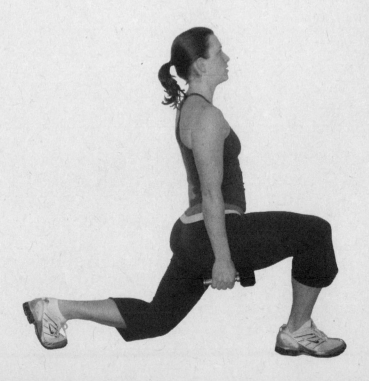

Hamstring Ball Roll

Target area

Back upper legs (hamstrings)

Equipment needed

Exercise ball, exercise mat

Set-up

Lie on your back on the mat with your bum at the edge and your heels on top of the exercise ball. Place your hands at your sides, palms down. Contract your abdominal muscles. Lift your hips off the floor so that only your shoulders, upper back, and hands are touching the floor.

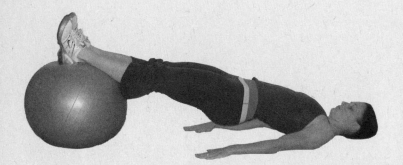

Movement

With your heels pressing into the ball, draw it in toward your bum, bending your knees as you do so. Pause once your heels are close to your bum, then straighten to starting position. Exhale as you draw the ball and your heels toward your bum, and inhale as you straighten your legs. Repeat for 12 repetitions to complete one set.

Tip

Keep your thighs squeezing together throughout the exercise to hold your balance on the exercise ball. Draw your heels toward your bum as close as you can.

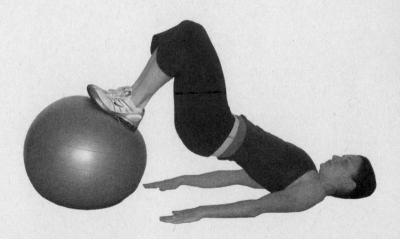

Calf Raise, Both Feet Weighted

Target area

Lower legs (gastrocnemius, soleus)

Equipment needed

Dumbbell, bottom step of a staircase

Set-up

Stand with your feet slightly wider than shoulder width apart and the balls of your feet on the edge of the stair so that your heels drop over the edge. Stand tall in your upper body, your toes pointed forward. Use one hand to hold the handrail or rest on the wall of the stairwell, and hold the dumbbell in the other hand.

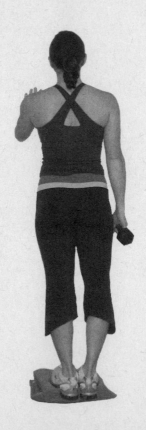

Movement

Contract your abdominal muscles. Slowly lift your body upward onto tip-toe. Hold for a moment, then slowly lower. Keep your back straight, one arm at your side with the dumbbell, the other hand holding the handrail. Exhale as you lift, and inhale as you lower. Repeat for 12 repetitions to complete one set. For your second set, place the dumbbell in the other hand.

Tip

Always hold the handrail or rest your hand on the wall while doing this exercise so that you don't fall back. You may need to stretch out the arch of your foot between sets.

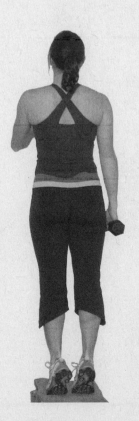

Weeks 4, 5, and 6: Core Exercises

Basic Crunch with Four-Count Pulse

Target area

Abdominals (rectus abdominis)

Equipment needed

Exercise mat

Set-up

Lie on your back on the mat with your knees bent and your feet flat on the floor. Clasp your hands lightly behind your head.

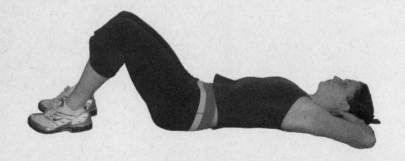

Movement

Contract your abdominal muscles to power you forward and slowly lift your head, neck, and shoulders off the mat. Your chin should be pointed forward, not tucked into your chest. Pause at the top, then pulse your upper body 1 inch (2.5 cm) forward and back four times. Slowly lower to resting position. Exhale as you lift, and inhale as you return to starting position, taking quick, short breaths during your 1-inch pulses. Repeat for 12 repetitions to complete one set.

Tip

Focus on a spot on the ceiling and lift your head, neck, shoulders, and chest up to it, keeping your chin off your chest.

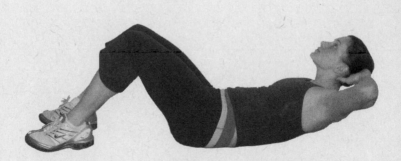

Side Bridge with Leg Lift

Target area

Sides of torso (quadratus lumborum, abdominal obliques)

Equipment needed

Exercise mat

Set-up

Lie on your side on the mat with your shoulders, hips, and legs aligned. Bend your knees at a right angle. Place your top arm on your hip, and the elbow of your bottom arm under your shoulders. The forearm of your bottom arm should be on the floor, and the upper part of this arm should support the shoulder.

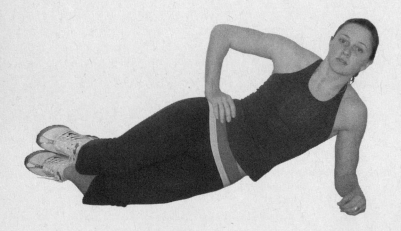

Movement

Contract your abdominal muscles and lift your hip off the mat. Your knees and bottom elbow should be on the floor supporting you. Slowly lift your top leg to hip height and straighten it. Hold for 10 to 15 seconds. If you find holding for 15 seconds easy, increase the time gradually. Keep your inhalation and exhalation fluid and rhythmical with deep breaths. Repeat on the other side to complete one set. Take a breath and rest 15 to 30 seconds, then move on to the next exercise.

Tip

When lifting your leg, keep it straight and long, with your foot flexed.

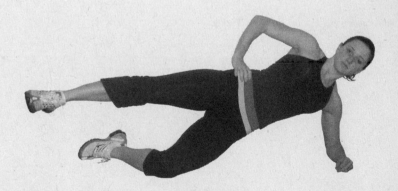

Women's Push-Up

Target area

Shoulders and torso

Equipment needed

Exercise mat

Set-up

Position yourself on all fours on the mat, with your hands slightly in front of your shoulders and slightly wider than shoulder width apart. Extend your arms straight, and lean forward to create a flat back. At this point, your arms should be straight and at a 90 degree angle to your body. Your knees are still on the mat, with your hips pushing

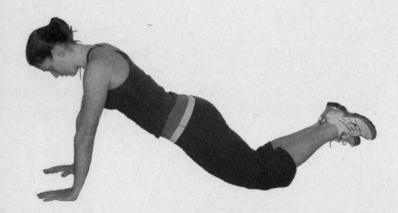

down toward it. Your body should be on an angle from your shoulders to your knees. This is the starting position.

Movement

Contract your abdominal muscles. Bend your arms, lowering your body toward the mat, until your face is nearly touching. Straighten your arms, pressing your body away from the mat. Inhale as you lower your body toward the mat, and exhale as you straighten your arms. Keep your body strong throughout the exercise. Repeat for 12 repetitions to complete one set.

Tip

Move your body as one unit.

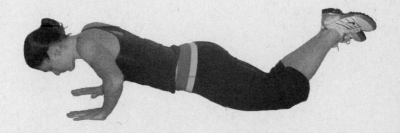

Weeks 7, 8, and 9: Upper Body

Chest Fly on Exercise Ball

Target area
Chest (pectorals major, pectorals minor)

Equipment needed
Dumbbells, exercise ball

Set-up
Sitting on the exercise ball, squeeze your buttocks and your thighs together and slowly walk your feet out so that your upper back, head, and neck are supported by the ball. Press your hips toward the ceiling so that your body is parallel to the floor. Keep squeezing your buttocks and thighs. With dumbbells in your hands, your palms facing inward, slowly extend your arms straight over your chest, over the midline of your body.

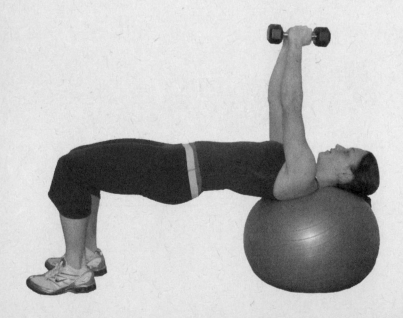

Movement

Contract your abdominal muscles and slowly lower your arms to your sides until you feel your upper arm touch the ball. During this movement keep your arms straight but not hyperextended, with your palms facing the ceiling. Pause, then slowly raise your arms back to starting position. Both arms are working at the same time and moving fluidly. Inhale as your arms move out wide, and exhale as you bring them back to starting position. Repeat for 12 repetitions to complete one set.

Tip

This exercise is a progression of the chest flys that you did in weeks 1, 2, and 3. Weeks 4, 5, and 6 add the exercise ball, to get you using your core. You may find that you cannot use much weight at first. Gradually add the weight you used when you did the exercise on the floor. Keep your back strong by pressing your hips toward the ceiling throughout the exercise.

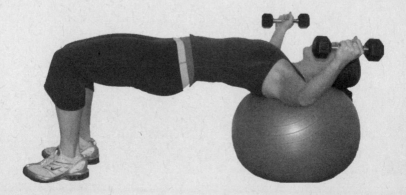

Seated Forward Row

Target area

Upper back (trapezius, rhomboids)

Equipment needed

Dumbbells or resistance band, exercise mat

Set-up

Sit on the mat with your legs in front of you, feet flexed so that your toes are pointing toward the ceiling. Sit up tall, with a flat back. Place the band around your feet and grip one end of the band in each hand. Hold your arms outstretched at shoulder height. If you use dumbbells for this exercise, keep your palms facing inward.

Movement

Contract your abdominal muscles and slowly draw your shoulder blades together. Your arms should brush at your sides, bending to

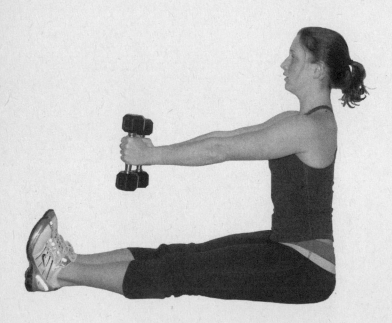

90 degrees. This calls for a very small movement in your upper back. If you are not feeling like your upper back is working by the 6th repetition, grasp the band lower down to increase the resistance, or increase the weight of the dumbbells. Exhale as you squeeze, and inhale as you release to starting position. Repeat for 12 repetitions to complete one set.

Tip

The movement in this exercise is in the shoulders. Although it is a very small movement, it is crucial to good posture—especially important for desk jockeys. Sit up tall and let your upper back do the work, as if you were rowing a boat. Trina recommends using resistance bands rather than dumbbells for this exercise. If you are holding dumbbells, the extra weight may tire your arms and not effectively work your upper back muscles.

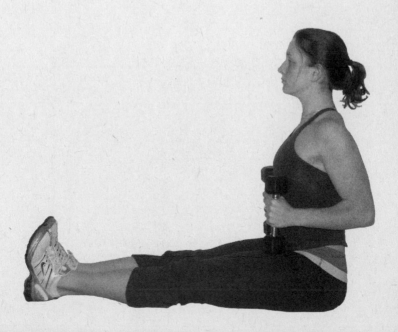

Chest Squeeze

Target area

Upper back (trapezius, latissimus dorsi)

Equipment needed

Dumbbells, exercise ball or chair

Set-up

Sit upright on the exercise ball or chair, feet flat on the floor and your back straight. Your shoulders should be directly over your hips. Hold one dumbbell in each hand above shoulder height, palms facing forward, your elbows at the height of your shoulders and bent at a 90 degree angle.

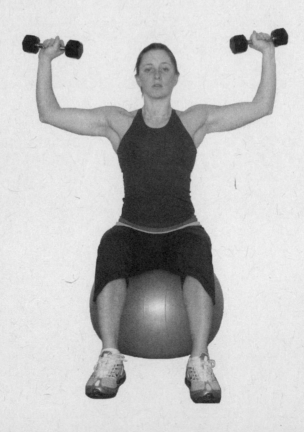

Movement

Contract your abdominal muscles. Slowly squeeze your forearms together in front of your body. Try to get your elbows as close together as possible. Pause, then open your arms to starting position. Keep your elbows at shoulder height. Exhale as you squeeze, and inhale as you open your arms. Repeat for 12 repetitions to complete one set.

Tip

Your elbows are going to want to creep below your shoulders, so watch for this. This exercise is best done in front of the mirror, so you can keep an eye on your alignment.

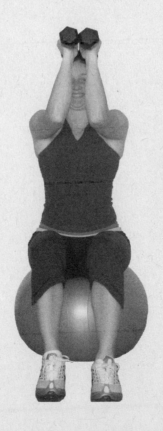

Bent Over Fly

Target area
Upper back (trapezius, rhomboid major, rhomboid minor)

Equipment needed
Dumbbells

Set-up
Stand with your feet slightly wider than shoulder width apart, your legs straight and one dumbbell in each hand. Bend forward from your hips until your torso is parallel to the floor and your arms are hanging straight down from your chest toward the floor. Keep your arms straight but not hyperextended, and your palms facing inward.

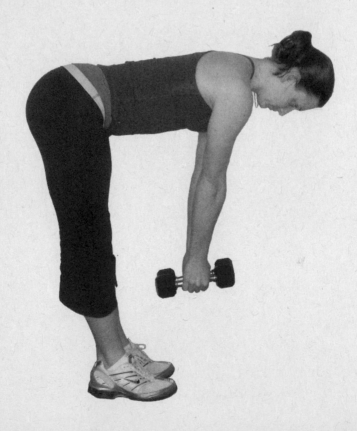

Movement

Contract your abdominal muscles. Lift your arms sideways and toward the ceiling, stopping at shoulder height. Palms face the floor. Pause, then slowly lower your arms to starting position. Exhale as you lift, and inhale as you lower. Repeat for 12 repetitions to complete one set.

Tip

Keep your core strong and your upper body parallel to the floor. This is a good exercise for your posture.

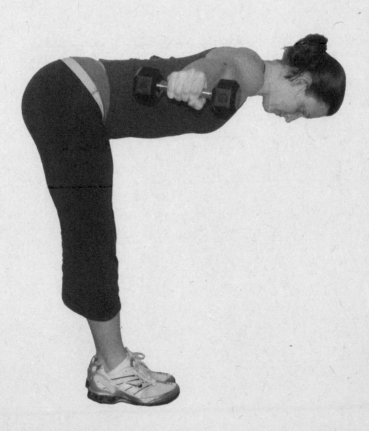

Weeks 7, 8, and 9: Lower Body

Basic Squat with Bicep Curls

Target area

Upper legs (quadriceps and hamstrings) and biceps

Equipment needed

Dumbbells

Set-up

Stand tall in your upper body, your feet slightly wider than shoulder width apart. Keep your toes pointed forward. Hold one dumbbell in each hand, palms facing forward.

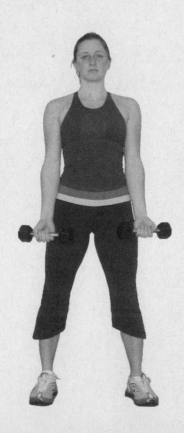

Movement

Contract your abdominal muscles. Keeping your upper body strong, bend your knees and slowly lower your body until your thighs are stopping when your elbows are overtop your knees and the dumbbells are at your shoulders. Pause at the bottom of your squat, then slowly rise as you straighten your arms. Inhale as you lower, and exhale as you rise. Control your movement throughout the exercise. Your upper body will lean forward but only slightly. Repeat for 12 repetitions to complete one set.

Tip

This exercise is primarily about leg strength. If the bicep curl is too much for you, keep the dumbbells at your sides.

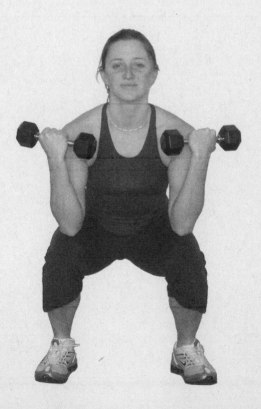

Walking Forward Lunge

Target area

Legs (quadriceps, hamstrings, calves)

Equipment needed

None

Set-up

Stand tall in your upper body, your feet close together. Contract your abdominal muscles. Take a giant step forward, placing one foot in front of you, knee bent. This is your static lunge position, from week 1.

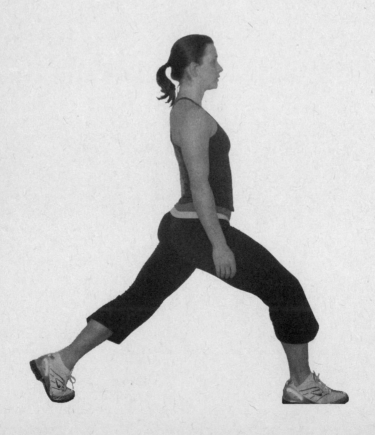

Movement

Slowly bend your back knee under your body. Your front knee bends but does not extend past the toes. Lower yourself in the lunge until you feel a stretch in the front of the thigh of the leg that is behind. Keep your arms resting at your sides. Pause, then slowly rise back up. With the leg that is stretched behind, take a giant step forward past your front leg. The leg that was behind is now in front. Exhale as you lower, and inhale as you rise. Repeat the movement with your other leg in front. Once both legs have taken a step, you have completed 1 repetition. Repeat for 12 repetitions to complete one set.

Tip

You cover a lot of distance with this exercise, so do it in a hallway. Remember to keep your back heel off the floor as you lower your body in the lunge.

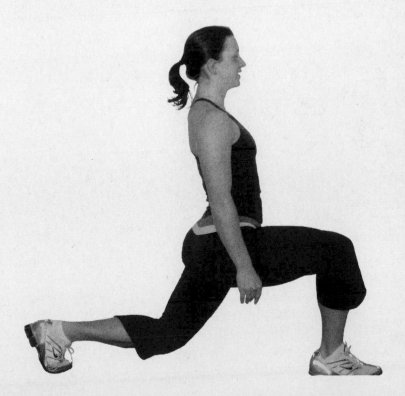

Hamstring Ball Roll with Four-Count Pause

Target area
Back upper legs (hamstrings)

Equipment needed
Exercise ball, exercise mat

Set-up
Lie on your back on the mat with your bum at the edge and your heels on top of the exercise ball. Place your hands at your sides, palms down. Contract your abdominal muscles. Lift your hips off the floor so that only your shoulders, upper back, and hands are touching the floor.

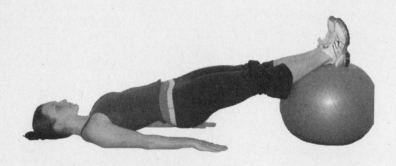

Movement
With your heels pressing into the ball, draw it toward your bum, bending your knees as you do so. Straighten to starting position. Exhale as you draw the ball and your heels toward your bum, and inhale as you straighten your legs. Lift one leg 1 inch (2.5 cm) off the ball. Hold for four counts as you take short quick breaths, inhaling and exhaling on each count of the hold. Place your leg back on the ball, draw the ball and your heels toward your bum, return to starting position, and lift your other leg 1 inch (2.5 cm) for four counts. Repeat for 12 repetitions to complete one set.

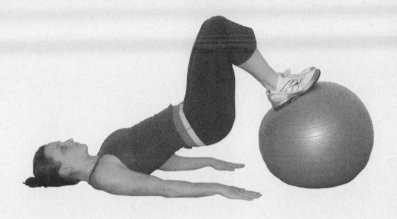

Tip

If you find it too difficult to pause for four counts, skip the pause.
Move your leg back to the ball without the pause.

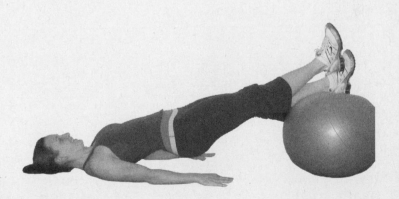

Single Calf Raise

Target area
Lower legs (gastrocnemius, soleus)

Equipment needed
Rolled-up bath towel or bottom step of a staircase

Set-up
Stand with the ball of one foot on the edge of the stair or towel roll so that your heel drops over the edge. Slightly bend your other leg, keeping it close to your standing leg. The foot of this leg should not be touching the stair or towel. Stand tall in your upper body, your toes pointed forward. Always hold the handrail or rest your hand on the wall for support.

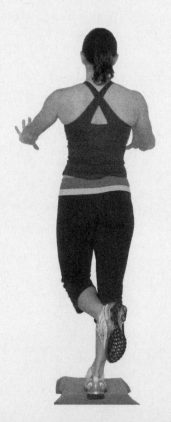

Movement

Contract your abdominal muscles. Slowly lift your body upward onto tip-toe. Hold for a moment, then slowly lower. Keep your back straight, one hand holding the handrail. Exhale as you lift, and inhale as you lower. Change leg and repeat 12 times to complete one set.

Tip

In this exercise you are bearing your full weight on one foot. You may need to stretch out your arch between sets.

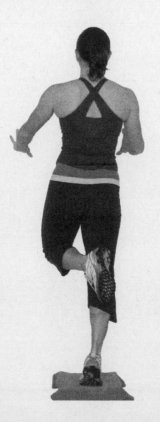

Weeks 7, 8, and 9: Core Exercises

Basic Crunch with Weight

Target area

Abdominals (rectus abdominis)

Equipment needed

Dumbbell, exercise mat

Set-up

Lie on your back on the mat with your knees bent and your feet flat on the floor. Place one dumbbell in both hands behind your head.

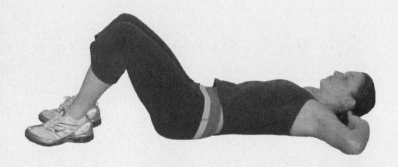

Movement

Contract your abdominal muscles to power you forward, slowly lifting your head, neck, shoulders, and the dumbbell off the mat. Keep your chin pointed forward, not tucked into your chest. Pause at the top of this movement, then slowly lower. Exhale as you lift, and inhale as you return to starting position. Repeat for 12 repetitions to complete one set.

Tip

If you find that adding the weight is too much for you, do the basic crunch without weight. Remember to keep your chin off your chest.

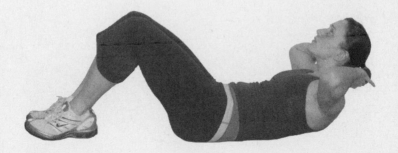

Straight Leg Side Bridge

Target area

Sides of torso (quadratus lumborum, abdominal obliques)

Equipment needed

Exercise mat

Set-up

Lie on your side on the mat with your shoulders, hips, and legs aligned, your legs stretched out. Place your top arm on your hip and the elbow of your bottom arm under your shoulder, your forearm on the mat.

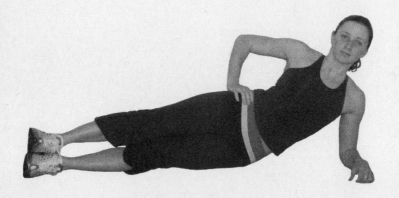

Movement

Contract your abdominal muscles and lift your hip off the mat. The outside edge of your bottom foot should be on the floor, supporting you along with your bottom arm. Hold for 10 to 15 seconds. If you find holding for 15 seconds easy, increase the time gradually. Keep your inhalation and exhalation fluid and rhythmical with deep breaths. Repeat on the other side to complete one set.

Tip

Keep both your legs straight, one on top of the other.

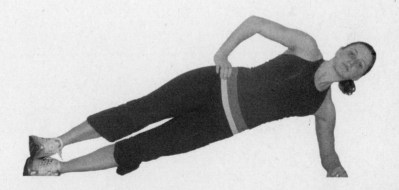

Women's Push-Up

Target area

Shoulders and torso

Equipment needed

Exercise mat

Set-up

Position yourself on all fours on the mat, with your hands slightly in front of your shoulders and slightly wider than shoulder width apart. Extend your arms straight and lean forward to create a flat back. At this point, your arms should be straight and at 90 degrees to your body. Keep your knees on the mat, your hips pushing down toward it.

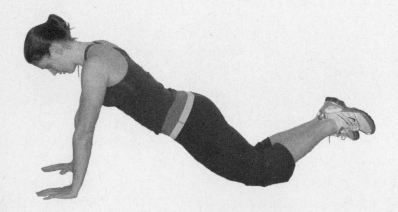

Your body should be at an angle from your shoulders to your knees. This is the starting position.

Movement

Contract your abdominal muscles. Bend your arms, lowering your body toward the mat, until your face is nearly touching. Straighten your arms, pressing your body away from the mat. Inhale as you lower your body toward the mat, and exhale as you straighten your arms. Keep your body strong throughout the exercise. Repeat for 12 repetitions to complete one set.

Tip

Move your body as one unit.

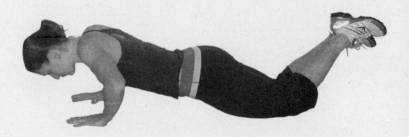

Weeks 10, 11, and 12: Upper Body

Bicep Concentration Curl

Target area
Front upper arms (biceps)

Equipment needed
Dumbbell

Set-up
Kneel on your left knee, your right foot flat on the floor in front of you. Take your right elbow and put it to the inside of your right knee. Hold one dumbbell in your right hand, palm facing outward. Put your left hand on your left hip.

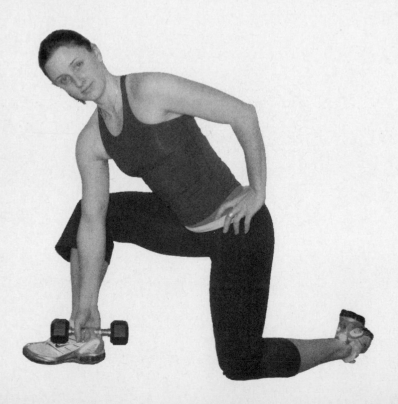

Movement

Contract your abdominal muscles. Curl your right arm, lifting the dumbbell toward your right shoulder. Pause at the top of this movement, then slowly lower. Exhale as you lift, and inhale as you lower. Repeat for 12 repetitions, then switch arms and repeat for another 12 to complete one set.

Tip

If you find the kneeling too hard on your knees, sit on a chair.

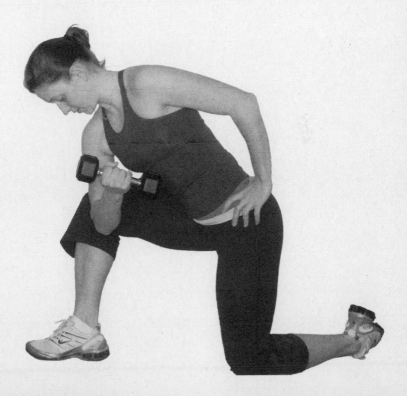

Triceps Dip

Target area

Back upper arms (triceps)

Equipment needed

Chair or bench

Set-up

With your back to a sturdy chair or bench, place your hands at the front edge of the seat, your fingers pointing forward and wrapped around the edge. Keep your legs outstretched in front of you, toes pointing toward the ceiling and your bum off the edge of the chair. At this point your arms are holding you up.

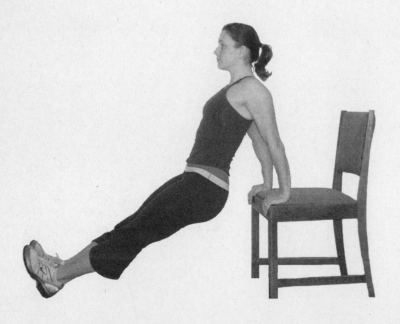

Movement

Contract your abdominal muscles. Slowly lower your bum to the floor by bending at your elbows. Lower to the point where your upper arm is parallel to the floor—no farther. Pause, then slowly rise to starting position. Control your movement throughout the exercise. Inhale as you lower, and exhale as you return to starting position. Repeat 12 times to complete one set.

Tip

If you find this movement too hard, bend your knees at a 90 degree angle with feet flat on the floor, instead of keeping your legs out straight.

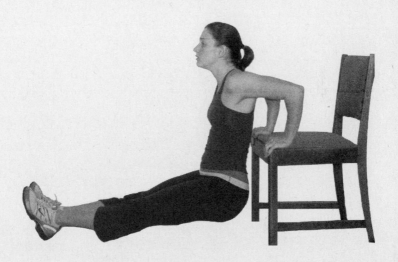

Lateral Lift

Target area
Shoulder rotator cuffs

Equipment needed
Dumbbells

Set-up
Stand tall in your upper body, your feet slightly wider than shoulder width apart and your knees slightly bent. Hold one dumbbell in each hand, your arms resting at your sides with palms facing inward.

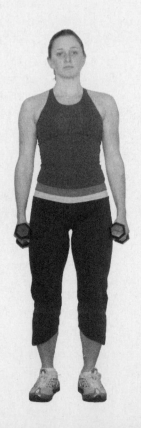

Movement

Contract your abdominal muscles and slowly raise your arms sideways to shoulder height. Pause, then slowly lower your arms. Exhale as you raise your arms, and inhale as you lower them to starting position. Continue to keep your abdominals squeezing tight to support your back and prevent it from arching. Repeat for 12 repetitions to complete one set.

Tip

Keep your shoulders down, away from your ears, and squeeze your abdominal muscles to keep your torso from moving.

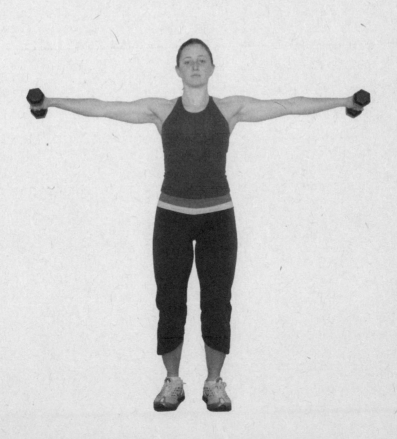

Anterior Lift

Target area
Shoulders

Equipment needed
Dumbbells

Set-up
Stand tall in your upper body, your feet slightly wider than shoulder width apart and your knees slightly bent. Hold one dumbbell in each hand, resting them on the front of your thighs with your palms facing inward.

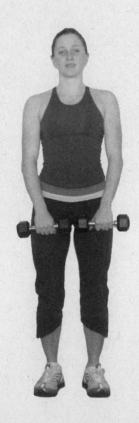

Movement

Contract your abdominal muscles. Slowly raise both arms in front of you to shoulder height. Pause, then slowly lower. Exhale as you raise your arms, and inhale as you lower them to starting position. Continue to keep your abdominals squeezing tight to support your back. Repeat for 12 repetitions to complete one set.

Tip

Do this exercise in front of a mirror so that you can see how high you are raising your arms. You don't want your arms to move above your shoulders. Keep your arms straight but not hyperextended.

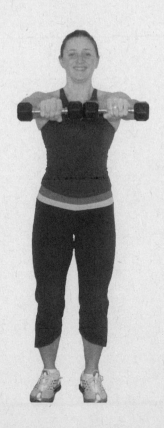

Weeks 10, 11, and 12: Lower Body

Basic Squat with Bicep Curls

Target area
Upper legs (quadriceps and hamstrings)

Equipment needed
Dumbbells

Set-up
Stand tall in your upper body, your feet slightly wider than shoulder width apart. Keep your toes pointed forward. Hold one dumbbell in each hand, palms facing inward.

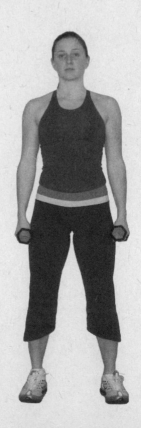

Movement

Contract your abdominal muscles. Keep your upper body strong, bend your knees and slowly lower your body until your thighs are almost parallel to the floor. As you bend your knees, start the bicep curls, stopping when your elbows are overtop your knees and the dumbbells are at your shoulders. Pause at the bottom of your squat, then slowly rise as you straighten your arms. Inhale as you lower, and exhale as you rise. Control your movement throughout the exercise: Your upper body will lean forward but only slightly. Repeat for 12 repetitions to complete one set.

Tip

This exercise is primarily about leg strength. If the bicep curl is too much for you, keep the dumbbells at your sides.

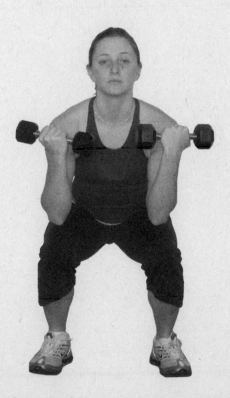

Walking Forward Lunge with Weight

Target area

Legs (quadriceps, hamstrings, calves)

Equipment needed

Dumbbell

Set-up

Stand tall in your upper body, your feet close together and one dumbbell in both hands resting on your thighs. Contract your abdominal muscles. Take a giant step forward, placing one foot out in front of you, knee bent. This is your static lunge position, from week 1.

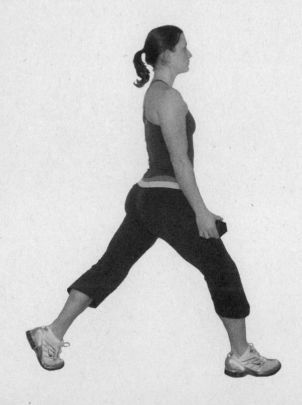

Movement

Slowly bend your back knee beneath your body. Your front knee bends but does not extend past the toes. Lower yourself in the lunge as you lift both your hands holding the weight to shoulder height. Lower yourself in the lunge until you feel a stretch in the leg that is behind. Pause, then slowly rise. Bring the dumbbell down to your thighs, and with the leg that is stretched behind you, take a giant step forward past your front leg. The leg that was behind is now in front. Exhale as you lunge, and inhale as you rise. Repeat with the other leg in front. Once you have worked both legs, you have completed 1 repetition. Repeat for 12 repetitions to complete one set.

Tip

Contracting your abdominal muscles will help you stay balanced. Do this exercise in a hallway, as you will be moving forward in big steps.

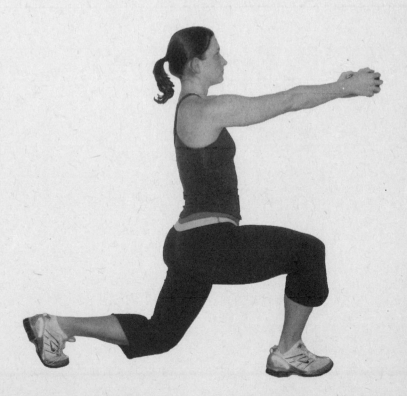

Dead Lift

Target area
Lower back, back upper legs (hamstrings, erector spine muscles)

Equipment needed
Dumbbells

Set-up
Stand tall in your upper body, your feet slightly wider than hip width apart. Rest your arms, one dumbbell in each hand, at your sides.

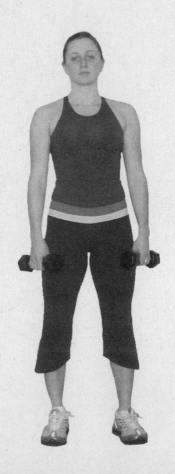

Movement

Contract your abdominal muscles. Bend forward from your hips so that your upper body folds over your lower body. Keep your legs straight and arms relaxed. Continue bending toward the floor until you are as close to it as you can get. Pause, then slowly return to standing. Inhale as you lower, and exhale as you return to starting position. Repeat for 12 repetitions to complete one set.

Tip

This exercise is most effective if it is done very slowly. Keep your legs straight so that you feel a stretch up the back of your legs, being careful not to hyperextend your knees. Keep your head and neck in a relaxed position.

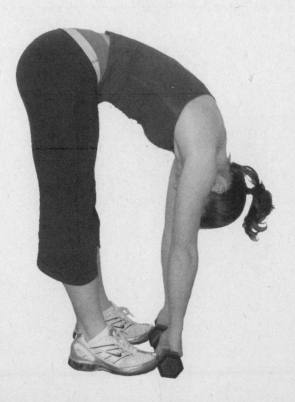

Single Calf Raise with Weight

Target area

Lower legs (gastrocnemius, soleus)

Equipment needed

Dumbbell, bottom step of a staircase, or rolled-up towel

Set-up

Stand with your feet slightly wider than shoulder width apart and the balls of your feet on a towel roll or the edge of the stair so that your heels drop over the edge. Stand tall in your upper body, keeping

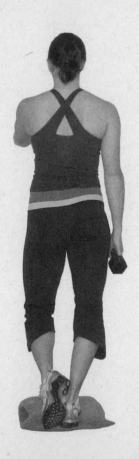

your toes pointed forward. Hold the handrail with one hand or rest your hand on the wall for support. Hold the dumbbell in your other hand. Lift the leg on the side that is not holding the dumbbell.

Movement

Contract your abdominal muscles. Slowly lift your body upward onto tip-toe. Hold for a moment, then slowly lower. Keep your back straight, one arm at your side, dumbbell in hand and the other hand holding the handrail. Exhale as you rise, and inhale as you lower. Repeat for 12 repetitions, then switch legs and repeat for another 12 to complete one set.

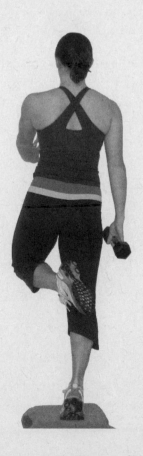

Weeks 10, 11, and 12: Core Exercises

Basic Crunch with Weight and Pulse

Target area

Abdominals (rectus abdominis)

Equipment needed

Dumbbell, exercise mat

Set-up

Lie on your back on the mat with your knees bent and your feet flat on the floor. Place one dumbbell in both hands behind your head.

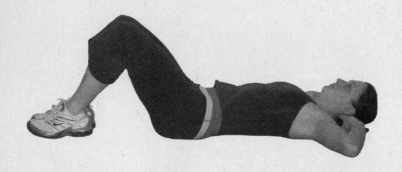

Movement

Contract your abdominal muscles to power you forward, slowly lifting your head, neck, shoulders, and the weight off the mat. Pulse your upper body four times, inching your upper body farther forward with each pulse. Slowly lower your body to resting position. Keep your chin pointed forward, not tucked into your chest. Exhale on the lift as you pulse forward, and inhale as you return to the mat. Repeat for 12 repetitions to complete one set.

Tip

This exercise is the basic crunch with weight that you did in weeks 7, 8, and, 9, now with pulses added. If you need to take out the pulses to complete your set, that's fine.

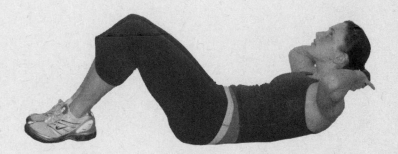

Straight Leg Side Bridge with Leg Lift

Target area
Sides of torso (quadratus lumborum, abdominal obliques)

Equipment needed
Exercise mat

Set-up
Lie on your side on the mat with your shoulders, hips, and legs aligned. Place your top arm on your hip, your elbow of your bottom arm under the shoulder. The forearm of your bottom arm should be on the floor.

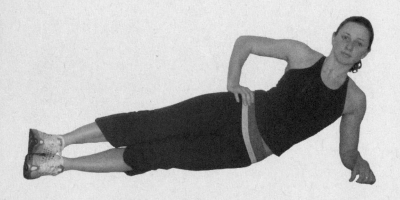

Movement

Contract your abdominal muscles and lift your hip off the mat. There are now two contact points with the floor: The outside edge of your bottom foot on the floor supporting you, along with the palm and forearm of your bottom arm. Raise your top leg off your bottom leg and hold at hip height for 10 to 15 seconds. If you find holding for 15 seconds easy, gradually increase the time. Keep your inhalation and exhalation fluid and rhythmical with deep breaths. Repeat on the other side to complete one set.

Tip

Keep both legs straight, one on top of the other. Lift the top leg no higher than your hip.

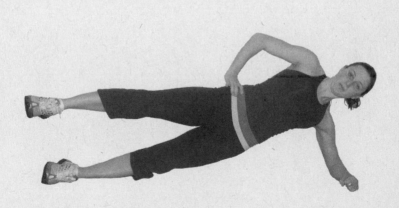

Full Push-Up

Target area
Shoulders and torso

Equipment needed
Exercise mat

Set-up
Lie face down on the mat with your palms down, slightly in front of your shoulders and slightly wider than shoulder width. Curl your toes under. Contract your abdominal muscles. Straighten your arms and lift your body off the mat.

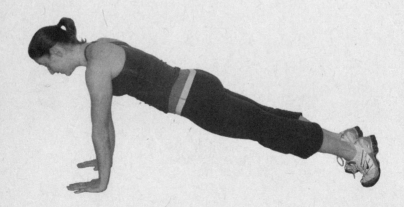

Movement

Keep your body in a straight position throughout the exercise. Bend your arms, lowering your body toward the mat until your face is nearly touching. Straighten your arms, pressing your body away from the mat. Inhale as you lower your body, and exhale as you return to starting position. Repeat for 12 repetitions to complete one set. Take a breath and rest 15 to 30 seconds before moving on to the next exercise.

Tip

You have now progressed from a half push-up (from the knees) to a full push-up. Drop back to your knees to complete the set if you need to.

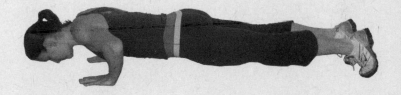

Stretching Exercises

The No-Fail 12-Week Fitness Program includes seven simple stretches to do after each cardiovascular workout, when your muscles are warm, to help prevent injuries. It's important that you stretch safely. Keep these tips in mind:

- Stretch slowly and smoothly without bouncing or jerking. Use gentle continuous movement or stretch-and-hold (for 10 to 30 seconds), whichever is right for the exercise.

- Focus on the target muscle that you're stretching. Relax the muscle and minimize the movement of other body parts.

- Stretch to the limit of the movement but not to the point of pain. Aim for a stretched, relaxed feeling.

- Don't hold your breath. Keep breathing slowly and rhythmically while holding the stretch.

Quadriceps Stretch

Set-up
Stand with one hand holding on to the back of a chair for balance. With your right leg, bend at the knee and draw your heel to your bum. Grasp your right ankle with your right hand. Stand tall in your upper body, your upper thighs together.

Stretch
Keep your left knee slightly bent. With your knees side by side and thighs together, hold your right heel close to your bum. You should feel a stretch in the front of your right thigh. For added stretch, push your hips slightly forward. Hold for a count of 10. Breathe deeply. Slowly release and switch sides. Do two times for each leg.

Tip

Keep your back tall and straight. Do not arch your back or push out your chest.

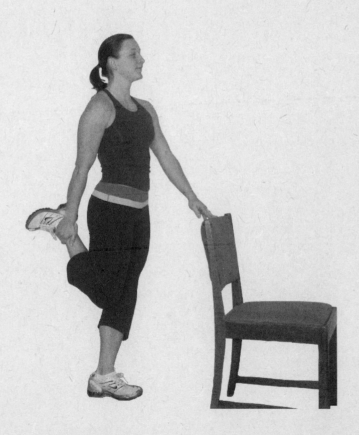

Hamstring Stretch

Set-up

Standing tall with your feet slightly wider than shoulder width apart, place your right heel on a chair seat, your toes pointed toward the ceiling. Keep both legs straight but not hyperextended.

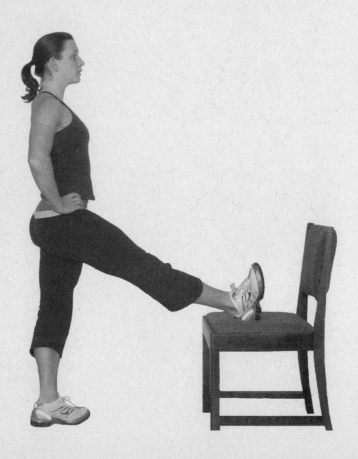

Stretch

Slowly bend forward from your hips until you feel a gentle tension in the back of the upper thigh of the leg that is on the chair. Hold for a count of 10. Breathe deeply. Slowly release and switch sides. Do two times for each leg.

Tip

As you bend forward, keep your hands on your hips and your chest pressing toward your toes.

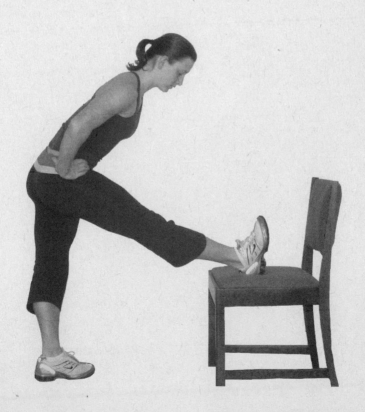

Lower Leg Stretch

Set-up

Standing tall with one hand on the back of a chair, place your other hand on your hip and stretch one leg out behind you as far as you can, keeping your heel on the floor.

Stretch

Bend your front leg slightly, until you feel a stretch in the calf of the leg that is stretched behind. Hold for a count of 10. Breathe deeply. Slowly release and switch legs. Do two times for each leg.

Tip

Do not let the knee of the front foot extend past the toes.

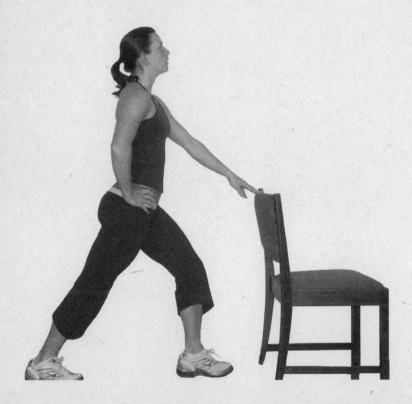

Triceps Stretch

Set-up

Standing tall with your feet slightly wider than shoulder width apart, place your right hand on your upper back, elbow pointed toward the ceiling. Place your left hand on your right elbow.

Stretch

Gently pull back on your right elbow so that your right hand reaches farther down your back. You will feel a stretch in your right back upper arm (triceps). Hold for a count of 10. Breathe deeply. Slowly release and switch arms. Do two times for each arm.

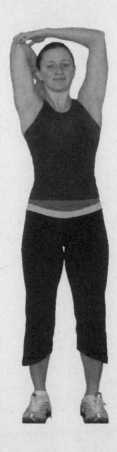

Tip

Make sure you are drawing your elbow back and not down into your shoulder joint. Keep your chin up, your head facing forward.

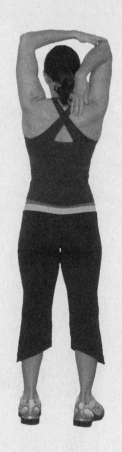

Shoulder Stretch

Set-up

Standing tall with your feet slightly wider than shoulder width apart, take your right arm and bring it across your body at shoulder height, your palm facing back. Place your left hand on your right elbow.

Stretch

Press your right arm closer to your chest so that you feel a stretch across your right upper shoulder. Hold for a count of 10. Breathe deeply. Slowly release and switch sides. Do two times for each arm.

Tip

Stand up tall and try not to twist your torso.

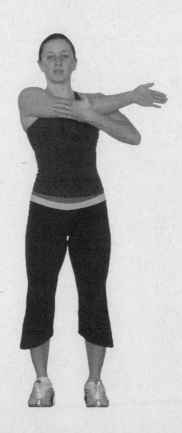

Upper Back Stretch

Set-up

Standing tall with your feet slightly wider than shoulder width apart, interlock your fingers in front of you. Raise your arms to shoulder height. Tuck your chin into your chest and turn your hands so that your palms face out.

Stretch

Push forward with your palms as you slowly round your upper back. Hold for a count of 10. Breathe deeply. Slowly release. Do two times.

Tip

Really round your back to get a good stretch.

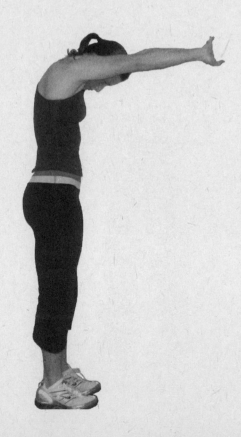

Chest Stretch

Set-up

Standing tall with your feet slightly wider than shoulder width apart, interlock your fingers behind your back. Squeeze your shoulder blades together.

Stretch

Slowly lift your arms away from your body behind your back. Hold for a count of 10. Breathe deeply. Slowly release. Repeat two times.

Tip

Keep your gaze straight ahead.

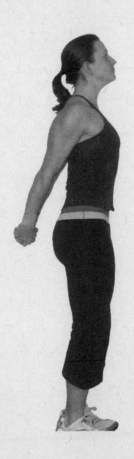

Putting It All Together: The No-Fail 12-Week Fitness Program

Week 1

Cardiovascular Workouts

Four

- Standard Cardio: Two (15 minutes each)
- Interval Cardio: One (18 minutes)

    Warm-up: 5 minutes

    Work phase: 1 minute at level 8 RPE or 80% maximum heart rate (HR)

    Recovery phase: 1 minute at level 6 RPE or 60% maximum HR

    Repeat work phase/recovery phase interval three times for a total of four intervals.

    Cool-down: 5 minutes

- Extended Cardio: One (22 1/2 minutes)

Stretching Sessions

Four; one after each cardio workout (5 minutes)

- Lower body: Quadriceps; Hamstring; Lower leg
- Upper body: Triceps; Shoulder; Upper back; Chest

Strength Workouts

Three times (30 minutes each)

- Upper body (two sets each): Bicep curl; Overhead triceps; Lat pull down; Chest fly
- Lower body (two sets each): Basic squat; Static forward lunge; Laying leg curl; Calf raise, both feet
- Core (two sets each): Basic crunch; Side bridge; Wall push-up

Week 2

Cardiovascular Workouts

Four

- Standard Cardio: Two (17 minutes each)
- Interval Cardio: One (18 minutes)

    Warm-up: 5 minutes

    Work phase: 1 minute at level 8 RPE or 80% maximum HR

    Recovery phase: 1 minute at level 6 RPE or 60% maximum HR

    Repeat work phase/recovery phase interval three times for a total of four intervals

    Cool-down: 5 minutes

- Extended Cardio: One (25 1/2 minutes)

Stretching Sessions

Four; after each cardio workout (5 minutes)

- Lower body: Quadriceps; Hamstring; Lower leg
- Upper body: Triceps; Shoulder; Upper back; Chest

Strength Workouts

Three (30 minutes each)

- Upper body (two sets each): Bicep curl; Overhead triceps; Lat pull down; Chest fly
- Lower body (two sets each): Basic squat; Static forward lunge; Laying leg curl; Calf raise, both feet
- Core (two sets each): Basic crunch; Side bridge; Wall push-up

Week 3

Cardiovascular Workouts

Four

- Standard Cardio: Two (19 minutes each)
- Interval Cardio: One (18 minutes)

    Warm-up: 5 minutes

    Work phase: 1 minute at level 8 RPE or 80% maximum HR

    Recovery phase: 1 minute at level 6 RPE or 60% maximum HR

    Repeat work phase/recovery phase interval three times for a
      total of four intervals

    Cool-down: 5 minutes
- Extended Cardio: One (28 1/2 minutes)

Stretching Sessions

Four; after each cardio workout (5 minutes)

- Lower body: Quadriceps; Hamstring; Lower leg
- Upper body: Triceps; Shoulder; Upper back; Chest

Strength Workouts

Three (30 minutes each)

- Upper body (two sets each): Bicep curl; Overhead triceps; Lat
  pull down; Chest fly
- Lower body (two sets each): Basic squat; Static forward lunge;
  Laying leg curl; Calf raise, both feet
- Core (two sets each): Basic crunch; Side bridge; Wall push-up

Week 4

For the next 3 weeks, you will do different strength and interval exercises. Detailed descriptions of each are given earlier in the chapter. Is it time to increase the weight of your dumbbells? Remember, strength exercises should feel difficult after 10 to 12 repetitions.

Cardiovascular Workouts

Four

- Standard Cardio: Two (21 minutes each)
- Interval Cardio: One (20 minutes)

    Warm-up: 5 minutes

    Work phase: 1 1/2 minutes at level 8 RPE or 80% maximum HR

    Recovery phase: 1 minute at level 6 RPE or 60% maximum HR

    Repeat work phase/recovery phase interval three times for a
        total of four intervals

    Cool-down: 5 minutes

- Extended Cardio: One (31 1/2 minutes)

Stretching Sessions

Four; after each cardio workout (5 minutes)

- Lower body: Quadriceps; Hamstring; Lower leg
- Upper body: Triceps; Shoulder; Upper back; Chest

Strength Workouts

Three (30 minutes)

- Upper body (two sets each): Hammer curl; Triceps kickback;
  Chest press; Standing forward row
- Lower body (two sets each): Basic squat with weights; Static
  forward lunge with weights; Hamstring ball roll; Calf raise, both
  feet weighted

- Core (two sets each): Basic crunch with four-count pulse; Side bridge with leg lift; Women's push-up

Week 5

Cardiovascular Workouts

Four

- Standard Cardio: Two (23 minutes each)
- Interval Cardio: One (20 minutes)

     Warm-up: 5 minutes

     Work phase: 1 1/2 minutes at level 8 RPE or 80% maximum HR

     Recovery phase: 1 minute at level 6 RPE or 60% maximum HR

     Repeat work phase/recovery phase interval three times for a total of four intervals

     Cool-down: 5 minutes

- Extended Cardio: One (34 1/2 minutes)

Stretching Sessions

Four; after each cardio workout (5 minutes)

- Lower body: Quadriceps; Hamstring; Lower leg
- Upper body: Triceps; Shoulder; Upper back; Chest

Strength Workouts

Three (30 minutes)

- Upper body (two sets each): Hammer curl; Triceps kickback; Chest press; Standing forward row
- Lower body (two sets each): Basic squat with weights; Static forward lunge with weights; Hamstring ball roll; Calf raise, both feet weighted

- Core (two sets each): Basic crunch with four-count pulse; Side bridge with leg lift; Women's push-up

Week 6

Cardiovascular Workouts

Four

- Standard Cardio: Two (25 minutes each)
- Interval Cardio: One (20 minutes)

  Warm-up: 5 minutes

  Work phase: 1 1/2 minutes at level 8 RPE or 80% maximum HR

  Recovery phase: 1 minute at level 6 RPE or 60% maximum HR

  Repeat work phase/recovery phase interval three times for a total of four intervals

  Cool-down: 5 minutes

- Extended Cardio: One (37 1/2 minutes)

Stretching Sessions

Four; after each cardio workout (5 minutes)

- Lower body: Quadriceps; Hamstring; Lower leg
- Upper body: Triceps; Shoulder; Upper back; Chest

Strength Workouts

Three (30 minutes)

- Upper body (two sets each): Hammer curl; Triceps kickback; Chest press; Standing forward row
- Lower body (two sets each): Basic squat with weights; Static forward lunge with weights; Hamstring ball roll; Calf raise, both feet weighted

- Core (two sets each): Basic crunch with four-count pulse; Side bridge with leg lift; Women's push-up

Week 7

For the next 3 weeks, you will do a new set of strength and interval exercises. Detailed descriptions of each are given earlier in the chapter. Is it time to increase the weight of your dumbbells? Remember, strength exercises should feel difficult after 10 to 12 repetitions.

Cardiovascular Workouts

Four

- Standard Cardio: Two (27 minutes each)
- Interval Cardio: One (22 minutes)

    Warm-up: 5 minutes

    Work phase: 2 minutes at level 8 RPE or 80% maximum HR

    Recovery phase: 1 minute at level 6 RPE or 60% maximum HR

    Repeat work phase/recovery phase interval three times for a total of four intervals

    Cool-down: 5 minutes

- Extended Cardio: One (40 1/2 minutes)

Stretching Sessions

Four; after each cardio workout (5 minutes)

- Lower body: Quadriceps; Hamstring; Lower leg
- Upper body: Triceps; Shoulder; Upper back; Chest

Strength Workouts

Three (30 minutes)

- Upper body (two sets each): Chest fly on exercise ball; Seated forward row; Chest squeeze; Bent over fly

- Lower body (two sets each): Basic squat with bicep curls; Walking forward lunge; Hamstring ball roll with four-count pause; Single calf raise

- Core (two sets each): Basic crunch with weight; Straight leg side bridge; Women's push-up

Week 8

Cardiovascular Workouts

Four

- Standard Cardio: Two (29 minutes each)
- Interval Cardio: One (22 minutes)

  Warm-up: 5 minutes

  Work phase: 2 minutes at level 8 RPE or 80% maximum HR

  Recovery phase: 1 minute at level 6 RPE or 60% maximum HR

  Repeat work phase/recovery phase interval three times for a total of four intervals

  Cool-down: 5 minutes

- Extended Cardio: One (43 1/2 minutes)

Stretching Sessions

Four; after each cardio workout (5 minutes)

- Lower body: Quadriceps; Hamstring; Lower leg
- Upper body: Triceps; Shoulder; Upper back; Chest

Strength Workouts

Three (30 minutes)

- Upper body (two sets each): Chest fly on exercise ball; Seated forward row; Chest squeeze; Bent over fly

- Lower body (two sets each): Basic squat with bicep curls; Walking forward lunge; Hamstring ball roll with four-count pause; Single calf raise

- Core (two sets each): Basic crunch with weight; Straight leg side bridge; Women's push-up

Week 9

Cardiovascular Workouts

Four

- Standard Cardio: Two (31 minutes each)
- Interval Cardio: One (22 minutes)

    Warm-up: 5 minutes

    Work phase: 2 minutes at level 8 RPE or 80% maximum HR

    Recovery phase: 1 minute at level 6 RPE or 60% maximum HR

    Repeat work phase/recovery phase interval three times for a
        total of four intervals

    Cool-down: 5 minutes

- Extended Cardio: One (46 1/2 minutes)

Stretching Sessions

Four; after each cardio workout (5 minutes)

- Lower body: Quadriceps; Hamstring; Lower leg
- Upper body: Triceps; Shoulder; Upper back; Chest

Strength Workouts

Three (30 minutes)

- Upper body (two sets each): Chest fly on exercise ball; Seated forward row; Chest squeeze; Bent over fly

- Lower body (two sets each): Basic squat with bicep curls; Walking forward lunge; Hamstring ball roll with four-count pause; Single calf raise

- Core (two sets each): Basic crunch with weight; Straight leg side bridge; Women's push-up

Week 10

For the next 3 weeks, you will do different strength and interval exercises. Detailed descriptions of each are given earlier in the chapter. Is it time to increase the weight of your dumbbells? Remember, strength exercises should feel difficult after 10 to 12 repetitions.

Cardiovascular Workouts

Four

- Standard Cardio: Two (33 minutes each)
- Interval Cardio: One (21 minutes)

  Warm-up: 5 minutes

  Work phase: 2 minutes at level 8 RPE or 80% maximum HR

  Recovery phase: 45 seconds at level 6 RPE or 60% maximum HR

  Repeat work phase/recovery phase interval three times for a total of four intervals

  Cool-down: 5 minutes

- Extended Cardio: One (49 1/2 minutes)

Stretching Sessions

Four; after each cardio workout (5 minutes)

- Lower body: Quadriceps; Hamstring; Lower leg
- Upper body: Triceps; Shoulder; Upper back; Chest

Strength Workouts

Three (30 minutes)

- Upper body (two sets each): Bicep concentration curl; Triceps dip; Lateral lift; Anterior lift

- Lower body (two sets each): Basic squat with bicep curls; Walking forward lunge with weight; Dead lift; Single calf raise with weight

- Core (two sets each): Basic crunch with weight and pulse; Straight leg side bridge with leg lift; Full push-up

Week 11

Cardiovascular Workouts

Four

- Standard Cardio: Two (35 minutes each)

- Interval Cardio: One (21 minutes)

    Warm-up: 5 minutes

    Work phase: 2 minutes at level 8 RPE or 80% maximum HR

    Recovery phase: 45 seconds at level 6 RPE or 60% maximum HR

    Repeat work phase/recovery phase interval three times for a total of four intervals

    Cool-down: 5 minutes

- Extended Cardio: One (52 1/2 minutes)

Stretching Sessions

Four; after each cardio workout (5 minutes)

- Lower body: Quadriceps; Hamstring; Lower leg

- Upper body: Triceps; Shoulder; Upper back; Chest

Strength Workouts

Three (30 minutes)

- Upper body (two sets each): Bicep concentration curl; Triceps dip; Lateral lift; Anterior lift

- Lower body (two sets each): Basic squat with bicep curls; Walking forward lunge with weight; Dead lift; Single calf raise with weight

- Core (two sets each): Basic crunch with weight and pulse; Straight leg side bridge with leg lift; Full push-up

Week 12

Cardiovascular Workouts

Four

- Standard Cardio: Two (37 minutes each)

- Interval Cardio: One (21 minutes)

    Warm-up: 5 minutes

    Work phase: 2 minutes at level 8 RPE or 80% maximum HR

    Recovery phase: 45 seconds at level 6 RPE or 60% maximum HR

    Repeat work phase/recovery phase interval three times for a total of four intervals

    Cool-down: 5 minutes

- Extended Cardio: One (55 1/2 minutes)

Stretching Sessions

Four; after each cardio workout (5 minutes)

- Lower body: Quadriceps; Hamstring; Lower leg

- Upper body: Triceps; Shoulder; Upper back; Chest

Strength Workouts

Three (30 minutes)

- Upper body (two sets each): Bicep concentration curl; Triceps dip; Lateral lift; Anterior lift

- Lower body (two sets each): Basic squat with bicep curls; Walking forward lunge with weight; Dead lift; Single calf raise with weight

- Core (two sets each): Basic crunch with weight and pulse; Straight leg side bridge with leg lift; Full push-up

6

The No-Fail Diet Menu Plans

To help you implement the No-Fail Diet, I have translated the Level 2 Meal Plan (1400 calories) into a 6-week menu plan that gives you all the protein, fruits, vegetables, and whole grains you need each day. The recipes called for in the menu plan are included in Chapter 7, along with a nutritional analysis per serving. I realize it's often easier to open a box of breakfast cereal or make a sandwich than it is to prepare a recipe from scratch, so the menu plan includes many meals and snacks that don't require a recipe. For the salads and mixed greens, use any of the five salad dressing recipes provided in Chapter 7, or a commercial variety that is low in fat, or calorie-reduced. Now that you have six weeks' worth of daily menus, you can rotate them and continue to use them for weeks 9 through 12. (If you skipped Phase 1, the 2-Week Quick Start meal plan, you can mix up these daily menus and follow them for weeks 5 through 12.)

Don't feel you have to use the menu plan exactly as it's presented. You might not want to adhere to a 6-week schedule or even a 2-week menu. Feel free to pick and choose meal and snack ideas to add to your own repertoire of healthy meals. Just remember to substitute foods from the same food group and follow the serving sizes outlined for the calorie level of your meal plan. For example, you would replace 2/3 cup (150 ml) brown rice with 1 cup (250 ml) cooked pasta, since both equal 2 Starchy Food servings.

The menu plan below adheres to the 1400 calorie meal plan, or Level 2. If you're following a different calorie level, refer to the No-Fail Diet meal plans on page 94 to adjust your portion sizes.

You'll find the menu plan presented in two formats: a brief overview of each week's meal ideas, and a detailed day-by-day menu that includes portion sizes, snacks and, healthy eating tips. You'll find a nutrient breakdown of calories, protein, carbohydrates, fibre, fat, cholesterol, and sodium for each day. When creating the menu plan, I've ensured that your *average* daily calorie intake does not exceed 1400 (Level 2) and your fat intake does not exceed 30% of calories. (You will notice that some daily menus provide a little less than 1400 calories, and others provide slightly more. What matters is your overall weekly intake—your average daily intake is 1400 calories.) The menu plan provides plenty of vitamins and minerals; however I still recommend a daily multivitamin and mineral supplement. (See pages 82 to 84 for my recommendations for multivitamins and calcium and vitamin D supplements.)

Weekly Menu Plans at a Glance

Week 3 Menu Plan

	MONDAY	TUESDAY	WEDNESDAY	THURSDAY	FRIDAY	SATURDAY	SUNDAY
Breakfast	Bran cereal Yogurt Berries	Whole-grain toast Strawberry Sunrise Smoothie (p. 289)	Oatmeal Yogurt	Whole-grain cereal Banana Milk	Breakfast pita Yogurt Fruit juice	French Toast (p. 286) Berries Yogurt	Breakfast Omelet (p. 286) Toast Fruit juice
Lunch	Tuna Salad Pita	Mixed greens with chickpeas and feta Crispbread	Chicken Wrap Vegetable soup	Hearty Black Bean Soup (p. 290) Mixed greens Crispbread	Open-Faced Roast Beef Sandwich Veggie sticks Apple	Salmon Salad Milk	Chicken Pesto Pizza Mixed greens
Dinner	Lemon Chicken (p. 309) Brown rice Sautéed asparagus and red bell peppers	Tomato Herb Pasta with Turkey (p. 314) Mixed greens	Sesame Ginger Salmon (p. 298) Steamed Quinoa (p. 284) Steamed broccoli and cauliflower	Shrimp Stir-Fry (p. 299) Basmati rice	Lime Cilantro Halibut (p. 295) Mashed sweet potatoes Asparagus	Balsamic Maple Pork Tenderloin (p. 301) Wild rice Lemon Swiss Chard (p. 329)	Moroccan Chickpea Stew (p. 321) Mixed greens

Week 4 Menu Plan

	MONDAY	TUESDAY	WEDNESDAY	THURSDAY	FRIDAY	SATURDAY	SUNDAY
Breakfast	Cranberry Apple Granola (p. 283) Apple Yogurt	Poached egg with tomato Toast Fruit juice	Leslie's Overnight Muesli (p. 284)	Whole-grain cereal Banana and blueberries Milk	Friendly Flax Smoothie (p. 287) Toast	Waffle Strawberries Yogurt Fruit juice	Breakfast Burrito (p. 285) Fresh Fruit Salad (p. 287)
Lunch	Red Pepper Lentil Soup (p. 292) Whole-grain roll Mixed greens	Tuna and crackers Veggie sticks Yogurt	Chicken Wrap	Salmon Pasta Salad (p. 292) Spinach	Smoked Ham Wrap	Curried Chicken Salad Sandwich (p. 305) Vegetable soup Milk	Mixed greens with Marinated Tofu (p. 320) Crispbread
Dinner	Jerk Chicken (p. 308) Brown rice Steamed carrots and beans	Tofu Vegetable Stir-Fry (p. 324) Rice noodles	Beef Curry (p. 302) Whole-wheat pasta Mixed greens	Turkey Burger (p. 315) Mixed greens	Honey Ginger Tilapia (p. 294) Brown rice Sautéed snow peas and bell peppers	Teriyaki Beef Kabobs (p. 312) Sweet Potato Wedges (p. 330)	Turkey Chili (p. 317) Steamed vegetables

Week 5 Menu Plan

	MONDAY	TUESDAY	WEDNESDAY	THURSDAY	FRIDAY	SATURDAY	SUNDAY
Breakfast	Oat bran cereal Yogurt Berries	Whole-grain cereal Milk Fruit juice	Very Berry Smoothie (p. 289) Toast	Mixed fruit Cranberry Apple Granola (p. 283) Milk	Poached egg Toast Cantaloupe	Whole-grain cereal Yogurt Fresh Fruit Salad (p. 287)	Breakfast Egg Sandwich Fruit juice
Lunch	Hearty Chicken Noodle Soup (p. 291) Crackers	Veggie Sandwich Yogurt	Julienne Salad Whole-grain roll	Pork Souvlaki Mixed greens	Turkey Sandwich Vegetable soup	Bean soup Whole-grain roll	Open-Faced Tuna Melt Mixed greens Milk
Dinner	Citrus Soy Salmon (p. 294) Bok choy Couscous	Thai Peanut Chicken (p. 314) Veggie Stir-Fry (p. 331)	Herbed Pork Tenderloin (p. 306) Roasted potatoes Mixed greens	Tomato Herb Pasta with Veggie Ground Round (p. 325) Mixed greens	Salmon Burger (p. 297) Spinach Salad, with Poppy Seed Dressing (p. 333)	Chicken Fajitas (p. 303) Mixed greens	Whole-Grain Lentil Casserole (p. 328) Steamed broccoli and carrots

Week 6 Menu Plan

	MONDAY	TUESDAY	WEDNESDAY	THURSDAY	FRIDAY	SATURDAY	SUNDAY
Breakfast	Oatmeal Blueberries Milk	Whole-grain cereal Peach Milk	Peachy Delight Smoothie (p. 288) Toast	Boiled egg Toast Fruit juice	Whole-grain cereal Banana and blueberries Milk	Toast Banana Milk	Breakfast Omelet (p. 286) Toast Milk
Lunch	Turkey Wrap	Lentil Soup with Turkey Sausage (p. 291) Mixed greens	Grilled Chicken Salad Crispbread	Roast Beef Sandwich	Black bean or lentil soup Crackers Bell pepper strips	Mediterranean Tuna Salad Fruit	Open-Faced Salmon Sandwich Fresh Fruit Salad (p. 287)
Dinner	Cajun Fish (p. 293) Wild rice Steamed green beans Baked Tomato	Chicken Mango Stir-Fry (p. 304) Basmati rice	Veggie Burger Mixed greens	Citrus Mustard Trout (p. 293) Pepper and Snow Pea Sauté (p. 330) Roasted potatoes	Indian Yogurt Chicken (p. 308) Basmati rice Steamed spinach and carrots	Teriyaki Sirloin Steak (p. 313) Baked potato Grilled bell peppers and zucchini	Turkey Lasagna (p. 318) Caesar salad

Week 7 Menu Plan

	MONDAY	TUESDAY	WEDNESDAY	THURSDAY	FRIDAY	SATURDAY	SUNDAY
Breakfast	Breakfast pita Yogurt Berries	Oat bran cereal Milk	Cranberry Apple Granola (p. 283) Yogurt Banana and blueberries	Toast Banana	Whole-grain cereal Milk Fruit juice	Poached egg Toast Cranberry Swirl Smoothie (p. 287)	French Toast (p. 286) Fresh Fruit Salad (p. 287) Milk
Lunch	Greek Wrap	Chicken Salad Sandwich Spinach Salad	Hearty Black Bean Soup (p. 290) Mixed greens	Open-Faced Ham and Cheese Sandwich	Tuna Salad	Mexican Bean Salad (p. 320) Crispbread Veggie sticks with ranch dip	Open-Faced Salmon Sandwich Mixed greens
Dinner	Grilled turkey breast Steamed Quinoa (p. 284) Mixed greens	Maple Glazed Salmon (p. 296) Brown rice Steamed snow peas and carrots	Turkey Burrito (p. 316) Mixed greens	Sweet and Sour Tofu Stir-Fry (p. 323) Rice noodles Steamed greens	Orange Rosemary Chicken (p. 309) Wild rice Roasted Brussels sprouts	Sesame Soy Trout (p. 298) Baked potato Sautéed broccoli and bell peppers	Honey Mustard Chicken (p. 307) Brown rice Sautéed vegetables

Week 8 Menu Plan

	MONDAY	TUESDAY	WEDNESDAY	THURSDAY	FRIDAY	SATURDAY	SUNDAY
Breakfast	Oatmeal Yogurt	Toast Peachy Delight Smoothie (p. 288)	Whole-grain cereal Berries Milk	Poached egg Toast Fruit juice	Breakfast pita Fruit	Toast Banana Milk	Boiled egg Toast Fruit juice
Lunch	Salmon Pasta Salad (p. 292)	Open-Faced Ham Sandwich Mixed greens Milk	Hearty Black Bean Soup (p. 290) Crackers Mixed greens	Chicken Wrap Vegetable soup	Tuna on Mixed Greens	Salmon Sandwich	Vegetarian Chili (p. 326) Pita Spinach Salad
Dinner	Chickpea Burger (p. 319) Mixed greens	Honey Garlic Chicken (p. 306) Basmati rice Balsamic Roasted Asparagus (p. 329)	Cumin Citrus Pork (p. 305) Baked potato Sautéed vegetables	Sole with Gremolata Sauce (p. 299) Wild rice Steamed spinach and carrots	Chicken Fajitas (p. 303) Mixed greens	Vegetarian Chili (p. 326) Baked potato Mixed greens	Roast Chicken Breast with Vegetables and New Potatoes

The No-Fail Diet Daily Menu Plans

Week 3: Monday

Breakfast
* 1/2 cup (125 ml) bran cereal, topped with 1 tbsp (15 ml) ground flaxseed, 3/4 cup (175 ml or 175 g container) low-fat (1% MF or less) plain or flavoured yogurt, and 1 cup (250 ml) mixed berries
* Coffee, tea, or water

Leslie's tip: When buying yogurt, choose one with 1% MF or less. It is not necessary to buy one that is artificially sweetened. However, if you wish to avoid added sugars, you may choose a yogurt that contains artificial sweeteners such as Splenda (sucralose). (Personally, I find that yogurts without artificial sweeteners are more filling.) Of course, the healthiest way to eat yogurt is to buy it plain and top with your own fruit.

Morning snack
* 1/2 cup (125 ml) baby carrots with 2 tbsp (25 ml) hummus
* 1 to 2 cups (250 to 500 ml) water

Lunch
* Tuna Salad Pita: To 3 oz (90 g) water-packed light tuna, add 4 tsp (20 ml) low-fat mayonnaise and 1 tbsp (15 ml) chopped fresh dill; place in a 6 inch (15 cm) whole-wheat pita along with lettuce, sliced tomato, and shredded carrot
* 1 to 2 cups (250 to 500 ml) water

Afternoon snack
* Cranberry Swirl Smoothie (p. 287)

Leslie's tip: If a homemade smoothie is not convenient for your afternoon snack, substitute with 1 Fruit serving and 1 Milk and Milk Alternative serving of your choice.

Dinner
* Lemon Chicken (p. 309)
* 2/3 cup (150 ml) steamed brown rice
* 1 cup (250 ml) asparagus tips and red bell pepper strips sautéed in 2 tsp (10 ml) canola oil
* 1 to 2 cups (250 to 500 ml) water

Nutrient breakdown: 1386 cal, 88 g pro, 27 g total fat (3 g sat. fat), 223 g carb, 40 g fibre, 82 mg chol, 1288 mg sodium

Week 3: Tuesday

Breakfast
* 1 slice whole-grain toast with 1 1/2 tsp (7 ml) nut butter
* Strawberry Sunrise Smoothie (p. 289)
* Coffee, tea, or water

Leslie's tip: Choose a whole-grain bread that delivers 2 grams of fibre per slice. Look for a bread that has a whole-grain (e.g., whole wheat, whole rye) listed as the first ingredient.

Morning snack
* 3/4 cup (175 ml or 175 g container) low-fat (1% MF or less) plain or flavoured yogurt with 1 Fruit serving of your choice
* 1 to 2 cups (250 to 500 ml) water

Leslie's tip: Not everyone likes to eat yogurt plain. Keep in mind that many fruit-bottom and flavoured yogurts deliver 4 to 6 teaspoons (20 to 30 ml) of sugar per 175 gram tub. The sugar numbers listed on the label include both natural milk sugar and added sugars. Once you account for the naturally occurring sugar, you're usually left with 2 to 4 teaspoons (10 to 20 ml) of added sugars. Ideally, choose a yogurt that has no more than 18 grams of sugar and 2 grams of saturated fat per 175 grams. Look for a daily value for calcium of at least 20% per 175 grams.

Lunch
* 1 to 2 cups (250 to 500 ml) mixed greens topped with 2/3 cup (150 ml) chickpeas, 1 oz (30 g) feta cheese, assorted raw veggies, 1 tbsp (15 ml) sliced almonds, and 4 tsp (20 ml) low-fat dressing
* 3 slices whole-grain crispbread crackers (Ryvita or Wasa)
* 1 to 2 cups (250 to 500 ml) water

Afternoon snack
* 3 cups (750 ml) plain air-popped or light microwave popcorn
* 1 to 2 cups (250 to 500 ml) water

Dinner
* Tomato Herb Pasta with Turkey (p. 314)
* 1 to 2 cups (250 to 500 ml) mixed greens with 4 tsp (20 ml) low-fat dressing
* 1 to 2 cups (250 to 500 ml) water

Nutrient breakdown: 1495 cal, 77 g pro, 38 g total fat (12 g sat. fat), 226 g carb, 38 g fibre, 109 mg chol, 2006 mg sodium

Week 3: Wednesday

Breakfast
* 1/2 cup (125 ml) cooked oatmeal or 1 package instant unflavoured oatmeal
* 1 cup (250 ml) low-fat (1% MF or less) plain or flavoured yogurt with 2 tbsp (25 ml) dried cranberries and 1 tbsp (15 ml) sunflower seeds
* Coffee, tea, or water

Morning snack
* 1 Fruit serving of your choice with 1 oz (30 g) part-skim (20% MF or less) cheese
* 1 to 2 cups (250 to 500 ml) water

Lunch
* Chicken Wrap: Spread a 10 inch (25 cm) soft whole-wheat or flax tortilla with 2 tbsp (25 ml) tzatziki; add 3 oz (90 g) roasted chicken breast, sliced cucumbers, tomatoes, and green pepper strips; wrap up and enjoy
* 1 cup (250 ml) vegetable soup
* 1 to 2 cups (250 to 500 ml) water

Leslie's tip: When buying commercial soups, look for brands that have less than 600 milligrams of sodium per cup.

Afternoon snack
* 3/4 cup (175 ml) red and green pepper strips with 2 tbsp (25 ml) low-fat ranch dressing as dip
* 1 to 2 cups (250 to 500 ml) water

Dinner
* Sesame Ginger Salmon (p. 298)
* 2/3 cup (150 ml) Steamed Quinoa (p. 284)
* 1/2 cup (125 ml) each steamed broccoli and cauliflower
* 1 to 2 cups (250 to 500 ml) water

Leslie's tip: Quinoa, an ancient grain that originated in the Andean region of South America, is high in protein and a good source of fibre. You can find quinoa in the bulk section of most health food stores.

Nutrient breakdown: 1462 cal, 93 g pro, 41 g total fat (7 g sat. fat), 190 g carb, 25 g fibre, 144 mg chol, 2269 mg sodium

Week 3: Thursday

Breakfast
- 1/2 to 3/4 cup (125 to 175 ml) whole-grain cereal
- 1 small banana, sliced
- 1 cup (250 ml) skim or 1% milk, or calcium-enriched plain soy milk
- Coffee, tea, or water

Morning snack
- 3/4 cup (175 ml or 175 g container) low-fat (1% MF or less) plain or flavoured yogurt with 1 cup (250 ml) chopped fresh fruit
- 1 to 2 cups (250 to 500 ml) water

Lunch
- 1 1/2 cups (375 ml) Hearty Black Bean Soup (p. 290)
- 1 to 2 cups (250 to 500 ml) mixed greens with 4 tsp (20 ml) low-fat dressing
- Whole-grain crispbread crackers (e.g., 5 Finn Crisps or 3 Ryvita)
- 1 to 2 cups (250 to 500 ml) water

Afternoon snack
- Whole-Wheat Pita Chips (p. 287) with 2 tbsp (25 ml) hummus
- 1 to 2 cups (250 to 500 ml) water

Dinner
- Shrimp Stir-Fry (p. 299)
- 2/3 cup (150 ml) steamed basmati rice
- 1 to 2 cups (250 to 500 ml) water

Leslie's tip: Shrimp are an excellent source of protein and they're very low in fat. If you're worried about their cholesterol content, don't be. Although shrimp do contain cholesterol (about 175 milligrams per 3 oz/90 g serving), cholesterol in foods has little or no effect on most people's blood cholesterol. If your blood cholesterol is high, you need to reduce your intake of foods high in saturated and trans fats. (The No-Fail Diet is low in both of these "bad" fats.)

Nutrient breakdown: 1436 cal, 75 g pro, 23 g total fat (5 g sat. fat), 252 g carb, 44 g fibre, 144 mg chol, 2205 mg sodium

Week 3: Friday

Breakfast

- 1 breakfast-sized (4 3/4 inch/12 cm) whole-grain pita (look for the brands Pita Break and Dempsters) with 2 tsp (10 ml) sugar-reduced fruit spread and 1 1/2 tsp (7 ml) nut butter
- 3/4 cup (175 ml or 175 g container) low-fat (1% MF or less) plain or flavoured yogurt
- 1/2 cup (125 ml) unsweetened fruit juice
- Coffee, tea, or water

Morning snack

- 12 oz (350 ml) latte, made with skim or 1% milk, or calcium-enriched soy milk (order the medium or tall size at coffee shops) OR 1 Milk and Milk Alternative serving of your choice

Lunch

- Open-Faced Roast Beef Sandwich: 3 oz (90 g) lean roast beef, mustard or horseradish, lettuce, and sliced tomato on 1 slice whole-grain bread
- 1/2 to 1 cup (125 to 250 ml) celery and carrots sticks with 2 tbsp (25 ml) low-fat dip
- 1 Fruit serving of your choice
- 1 to 2 cups (250 to 500 ml) water

Afternoon snack

- 1 low-fat granola bar
- 1 to 2 cups (250 to 500 ml) water

Leslie's tip: Granola bars are a convenient, portable, and healthy snack—as long as they don't contain chocolate chips, candy pieces, or caramel and are not wrapped in a yogurt coating. Read labels when buying granola bars. Look for one that has at least 2 grams of fibre, zero grams of trans fat, and no more than 1 gram of saturated fat and 10 grams of sugar per serving. This snack should contain no more than 150 calories.

Dinner

- 3 oz (90 g) serving of Lime Cilantro Halibut (p. 295)
- 1/2 cup (125 ml) sweet potato, mashed with 2 tbsp (25 ml) orange juice
- 6 spears of asparagus, steamed or roasted
- 1 to 2 cups (250 to 500 ml) water

Nutrient breakdown: 1350 cal, 88 g pro, 31 g total fat (8 g sat. fat), 190 g carb, 23 g fibre, 101 mg chol, 1474 mg sodium

Week 3: Saturday

Breakfast
- French Toast (p. 286), topped with 1 cup (250 ml) mixed berries, 3/4 cup (175 ml or 175 g container) low-fat (1% MF or less) plain or flavoured yogurt, and a drizzle of maple syrup
- Coffee, tea, or water

Lunch
- Salmon Salad: 1 to 2 cups (250 to 500 ml) mixed greens topped with 3 oz (90 g) canned salmon, 2 tsp (10 ml) low-fat dressing, and 1 tbsp (15 ml) cashews; add 1 cup (250 ml) assorted chopped vegetables (peppers, mushrooms, tomatoes)
- 1 cup (250 ml) skim or 1% milk, or calcium-enriched plain soy milk

Afternoon snack
- 1 energy bar (no more than 200 calories)
- 1 to 2 cups (250 to 500 ml) water

Leslie's tip: When shopping for energy bars, read the labels. Avoid energy bars made with hydrogenated oils, palm kernel oil, or coconut oil. Choose a bar with 20 to 25 grams carbohydrate, at least 3 grams of fibre, and no more than 2 grams of saturated fat.

Dinner
- 3 oz (90 g) serving of Balsamic Maple Pork Tenderloin (p. 301)
- 2/3 cup (150 ml) steamed wild rice
- Lemon Swiss Chard (p. 329)
- 1 to 2 cups (250 to 500 ml) water

Nutrient breakdown: 1393 cal, 82 g pro, 38 g total fat (9 g sat. fat), 191 g carb, 20 g fibre, 272 mg chol, 1247 mg sodium

Week 3: Sunday

Breakfast
- Breakfast Omelet (p. 286)
- 1 slice whole-grain toast with 1 tsp (5 ml) butter or non-hydrogenated margarine
- 1/2 cup (125 ml) unsweetened fruit juice
- Coffee, tea, or water

Lunch
- Chicken Pesto Pizza: Spread a 10 inch (25 cm) soft whole-grain tortilla with 1 tbsp (15 ml) pesto sauce and top with 1 1/2 oz (45 g) crumbed goat cheese, 2 oz (60 g) chopped chicken breast, and 2 tbsp (25 ml) chopped sun-dried tomatoes; bake at 425°F (220°C) for 8 to 10 minutes
- 1 to 2 cups (250 to 500 ml) mixed greens with fresh lemon juice or seasoned rice vinegar as dressing
- 1 to 2 cups (250 to 500 ml) water

Afternoon snack
- Peachy Delight Smoothie (p. 288)

Leslie's tip: If a homemade smoothie is not convenient for your afternoon snack, substitute with 1 Fruit serving and 1 Milk and Milk Alternative serving of your choice.

Dinner
- Moroccan Chickpea Stew (p. 321)
- 1 to 2 cups (250 to 500 ml) mixed greens with 4 tsp (20 ml) low-fat dressing
- 1 to 2 cups (250 to 500 ml) water

Nutrient breakdown: 1354 cal, 76 g pro, 46 g total fat (17 g sat. fat), 167 g carb, 22 g fibre, 467 mg chol, 2267 mg sodium

Week 4: Monday

Breakfast
- 1/3 cup (75 ml) Cranberry Apple Granola (p. 285), topped with 1 chopped medium apple and 3/4 cup (175 ml or 175 g container) low-fat (1% MF or less) plain or flavoured yogurt
- Coffee, tea, or water

Leslie's tip: The recipe for Cranberry Apple Granola makes 18 Starchy Food servings (1 serving equals 1/3 cup/75 ml). Store granola in the fridge and use anytime in place of other starchy foods outlined in the No-Fail Diet Menu Plan. Remember, this meal plan is flexible—you are free to follow it exactly, or substitute other foods whenever you wish. Just be sure to stick to the serving sizes outlined on your No-Fail Diet Meal Plan (see page 94).

Morning snack
- 12 oz (350 ml) latte, made with skim or 1% milk, or calcium-enriched soy milk (order the medium or tall size in coffee shops) OR 1 Milk and Milk Alternative serving of your choice

Lunch
- 1 1/2 cups (375 ml) Red Pepper Lentil Soup (p. 292)
- 1 small whole-grain roll (3 oz/90 g serving)
- 1 to 2 cups (250 to 500 ml) mixed greens with 4 tsp (20 ml) low-fat dressing
- 1 to 2 cups (250 to 500 ml) water

Afternoon snack
- 1 Fruit serving of your choice
- 10 plain, unsalted almonds
- 1 to 2 cups (250 to 500 ml) water

Dinner
- Jerk Chicken (p. 308)
- 2/3 cup (150 ml) steamed brown rice
- 1/2 cup (125 ml) each steamed carrots and green beans
- 1 to 2 cups (250 to 500 ml) water

Nutrient breakdown: 1396 cal, 74 g pro, 32 g total fat (5 g sat. fat), 217 g carb, 29 g fibre, 68 mg chol, 2059 mg sodium

Week 4: Tuesday

Breakfast
* 1 poached egg on 1 slice whole-grain toast with sliced tomato
* 1/2 cup (125 ml) unsweetened fruit juice OR 1 fruit serving of your choice
* Coffee, tea, or water

Morning snack
* 1 pear with 5 walnut halves
* 1 to 2 cups (250 to 500 ml) water

Lunch
* 2 oz (60 g) mini-can seasoned tuna on whole-grain crispbread crackers (3 Wasa or 6 Ryvita)
* 1 cup (250 ml) mixed raw veggie sticks
* 3/4 cup (175 ml or 175 g container) low-fat (1% MF or less) plain or flavoured yogurt
* 1 to 2 cups (250 to 500 ml) water

Afternoon snack
* 1 energy bar
* 1 to 2 cups (250 to 500 ml) water

Leslie's tip: Choose a bar with 7 to 15 grams of protein, 20 to 25 grams carbohydrate, at least 3 grams of fibre, and no more than 2 grams of saturated fat. For women, energy bars should be no more than 200 calories; for men no more than 250.

Dinner
* Tofu Vegetable Stir-Fry (p. 324)
* 1 cup (250 ml) cooked rice noodles
* 1 to 2 cups (250 to 500 ml) water

Nutrient breakdown: 1297 cal, 67 g pro, 37 g total fat (6 g sat. fat), 187 g carb, 28 g fibre, 207 mg chol, 1014 mg sodium

Week 4: Wednesday

Breakfast
- 1 cup (250 ml) Leslie's Overnight Muesli (p. 284)
- Coffee, tea, or water

Morning snack
- 3/4 cup (175 ml or 175 g container) low-fat (1% MF or less) plain or flavoured yogurt
- 1 to 2 cups (250 to 500 ml) water

Lunch
- Chicken Wrap: Place 3 oz (90 g) grilled chicken breast in a 6 inch (15 cm) pita pocket with spinach leaves, sliced tomato, shredded carrot, and 2 tbsp (25 ml) hummus
- 1 to 2 cups (250 to 500 ml) water

Afternoon snack
- 1 oz (30 g) part-skim cheese
- 1 Fruit serving of your choice
- 1 to 2 cups (250 to 500 ml) water

Dinner
- Beef Curry (p. 302)
- 1 cup (250 ml) whole-wheat pasta
- 1 to 2 cups (250 to 500 ml) mixed greens with 4 tsp (20 ml) low-fat dressing
- 1 to 2 cups (250 to 500 ml) water

Nutrient breakdown: 1347 cal, 94 g pro, 27 g total fat (6 g sat. fat), 195 g carb, 27 g fibre, 130 mg chol, 1747 mg sodium

Week 4: Thursday

Breakfast
- 1/2 to 3/4 cup (125 to 175 ml) whole-grain cereal topped with 1/2 sliced banana and 1/2 cup (125 ml) blueberries
- 1 cup (250 ml) skim or 1% milk, or calcium-enriched plain soy milk
- Coffee, tea, or water

Morning snack
- 7 dried apricot halves and 10 plain, unsalted almonds
- 1 to 2 cups (250 to 500 ml) water

Leslie's tip: A snack of dried apricots and almonds provides carbohydrate, protein, fibre, and iron. For convenience, prepackage apricots and almonds in snack-size zip-lock bags. Portioning out the snack ahead of time will also help prevent you from eating too many almonds.

Lunch
- Salmon Pasta Salad (p. 294) served on 2 cups (500 ml) raw spinach leaves
- 1 to 2 cups (250 to 500 ml) water

Afternoon snack
- 12 oz (350 ml) chai tea latte or regular latte, made with skim or 1% milk, or calcium-enriched soy milk OR 1 Milk and Milk Alternative serving of your choice

Leslie's tip: To reduce the sugar content of a coffee-shop chai tea latte, ask that it be made with half the usual amount of syrup. If you don't drink coffee or tea, try a "steamer" made with milk and a sugar-free vanilla shot.

Dinner
- Turkey Burger (p. 317) served in a 6 inch (15 cm) whole-grain pita with spinach leaves, sliced tomato and 1/8 of an avocado, sliced
- 1 to 2 cups (250 to 500 ml) mixed greens with 4 tsp (20 ml) low-fat dressing
- 1 to 2 cups (250 to 500 ml) water

Nutrient breakdown: 1433 cal, 84 g pro, 44 g total fat (11 g sat. fat), 204 g carb, 38 g fibre, 164 mg chol, 1726 mg sodium

Week 4: Friday

Breakfast
- Friendly Flax Smoothie (p. 288)
- 1 slice whole-grain toast with 1 tbsp (15 ml) reduced-sugar fruit spread
- Coffee, tea, or water

Morning snack
- 1/4 cup (50 ml) 1% MF or fat-free cottage cheese with 1/2 cup (125 ml) pineapple chunks
- 1 to 2 cups (250 to 500 ml) water

Leslie's tip: You can make this snack yourself or you can buy it ready-made in the dairy section of your grocery store. Try Nordica Single-Serve Cottage Cheese with peach, strawberry, or tropical fruit. Each 113 g serving has 110 calories, 11 grams of protein, 110 milligrams of calcium, and no more than 2 grams of fat.

Lunch
- Smoked Ham Wrap: Spread a 10 inch (25 cm) soft whole-wheat tortilla with honey Dijon mustard; add 2 oz (60 g) black forest ham, 1 oz (30 g) part-skim cheese, bell pepper strips, and lettuce
- 1 to 2 cups (250 to 500 ml) water

Afternoon snack
- 1/2 cup (125 ml) baby carrots with 2 tbsp (25 ml) tzatziki
- 1 to 2 cups (250 to 500 ml) water

Dinner
- 3 oz (90 g) serving of Honey Ginger Tilapia (p. 294)
- 2/3 cup (150 ml) steamed brown rice
- 1/2 cup (125 ml) snow peas and 1/2 cup (125 ml) red bell pepper strips, sautéed
- 1 to 2 cups (250 to 500 ml) water

Leslie's tip: Sauté or stir-fry vegetables in a non-stick pan, adding 1 tsp (5 ml) sesame oil at the end of cooking for a flavour boost.

Nutrient breakdown: 1405 cal, 62 g pro, 29 g total fat (8 g sat. fat), 213 g carb, 23 g fibre, 102 mg chol, 2299 mg sodium

Week 4: Saturday

Breakfast
- 1 whole-wheat homemade or toaster waffle topped with 3/4 cup (175 ml) sliced strawberries and 3/4 cup (175 ml or 175 g container) low-fat (1% MF or less) plain or flavoured yogurt
- 1/2 cup (125 ml) unsweetened fruit juice
- Coffee, tea, or water

Leslie's tip: When buying frozen waffles, choose a brand that is made with whole grains (e.g., whole-wheat flour, flaxseed, or oats) and contains no trans fat. Recommended brands include Nature's Path, Lifestream, and Van's.

Lunch
- Curried Chicken Salad Sandwich (p. 305)
- 1 cup (250 ml) vegetable soup
- 1 cup (250 ml) skim or 1% milk, or calcium-enriched plain soy milk
- 1 to 2 cups (250 to 500 ml) water

Afternoon snack
- 3 cups (750 ml) plain air-popped or microwave light popcorn
- 1 to 2 cups (250 to 500 ml) water

Dinner
- Teriyaki Beef Kabobs (p. 312)
- Sweet Potato Wedges (p. 330)
- 1 to 2 cups (250 to 500 ml) water

Nutrient breakdown: 1301 cal, 83 g pro, 29 g total fat (6 g sat. fat), 183 g carb, 22 g fibre, 119 mg chol, 1803 mg sodium

Week 4: Sunday

Breakfast
- Breakfast Burrito (p. 285)
- 1 cup (250 ml) Fresh Fruit Salad (p. 287)
- Coffee, tea, or water

Lunch
- 1 to 2 cups (250 to 500 ml) mixed greens with Marinated Tofu (p. 320)
- Whole-grain crispbread crackers (e.g., 3 Wasa or 6 Ryvita)
- 1 to 2 cups (250 to 500 ml) water

Afternoon snack
- Mango Tango Smoothie (p. 288)

Dinner
- Turkey Chili (p. 317)
- 1 cup (250 ml) steamed vegetables of your choice
- 1 to 2 cups (250 to 500 ml) water

Leslie's tip: The weekend is a great time to batch cook for your busy week ahead. Consider doubling the Turkey Chili recipe and freeze the extra in single-meal portions.

Nutrient breakdown: 1422 cal, 88 g pro, 38 g total fat (9 g sat. fat), 203 g carb, 35 g fibre, 256 mg chol, 1414 mg sodium

Week 5: Monday

Breakfast

* 1/2 cup (125 ml) hot oat bran cereal, topped with 1 tbsp (15 ml) ground flaxseed and 2 tbsp (25 ml) dried cranberries
* 3/4 cup (175 ml or 175 g container) low-fat (1% MF or less) plain or flavoured yogurt with 1/2 cup (125 ml) mixed berries
* Coffee, tea, or water

Morning snack

* 1 Fruit serving of your choice with 10 plain, unsalted almonds
* 1 to 2 cups (250 to 500 ml) water

Lunch

* Hearty Chicken Noodle Soup (p. 291)
* 7 whole-wheat soda crackers
* 1 to 2 cups (250 to 500 ml) water

Afternoon snack

* 12 oz (350 ml) green tea latte, made with skim or 1% milk, or calcium-enriched soy milk OR 1 Milk and Milk Alternative serving of your choice

Dinner

* Citrus Soy Salmon (p. 294)
* 1 cup (250 ml) steamed bok choy
* 2/3 cup (150 ml) whole-wheat couscous
* 1 to 2 cups (250 to 500 ml) water

Leslie's tip: Couscous is a light and fluffy grain made from semolina (coarsely ground durum wheat). To boost your intake of fibre and anti-oxidants, look for whole-wheat couscous, available in most grocery stores.

Nutrient breakdown: 1349 cal, 85 g pro, 42 g total fat (8 g sat. fat), 166 g carb, 27 g fibre, 142 mg chol, 2382 mg sodium

Week 5: Tuesday

Breakfast
* 1/2 to 3/4 cup (125 to 175 ml) whole-grain cereal with 2 tbsp (25 ml) raisins
* 1 cup (250 ml) skim or 1% milk, or calcium-enriched plain soy milk
* 1/2 cup (125 ml) unsweetened fruit juice
* Coffee, tea, or water

Morning snack
* 1 Fruit serving of your choice
* 1 oz (30 g) part-skim cheese
* 1 to 2 cups (250 to 500 ml) water

Lunch
* Veggie Sandwich: 2 tbsp hummus, 5 pecan halves, baby spinach leaves, sliced tomato, 1/8 avocado, and grated carrots on 2 slices whole-grain bread
* 3/4 cup (175 ml or 175 g container) low-fat (1% MF or less) plain or flavoured yogurt
* 1 to 2 cups (250 to 500 ml) water

Afternoon snack
* 2 oz (60 g) mini-can seasoned tuna with 7 whole-wheat soda crackers
* 1 to 2 cups (250 to 500 ml) water

Dinner
* Thai Peanut Chicken (p. 314)
* Veggie Stir-Fry (p. 331)
* 1 to 2 cups (250 to 500 ml) water

Leslie's tip: If you're short on time or don't feel like washing and chopping fresh vegetables, use frozen vegetables. My favourites are Europe's Best frozen vegetable medleys. Cook first for 2 minutes in a small amount of boiling water, then add them to your stir-fry and cook a few minutes longer. (Keep in mind that frozen vegetables cook faster than fresh ones.) Put any frozen vegetables not used immediately back in the freezer.

Nutrient breakdown: 1399 cal, 83 g pro, 38 g total fat (7 g sat. fat), 211 g carb, 39 g fibre, 80 mg chol, 1859 mg sodium

Week 5: Wednesday

Breakfast
- Very Berry Smoothie (p. 289)
- 1 or 2 slices whole-grain toast with 1 1/2 tsp (7 ml) nut butter
- Coffee, tea, or water

Morning snack
- 3/4 cup (175 ml or 175 g container) low-fat (1% MF or less) plain or flavoured yogurt
- 1 to 2 cups (250 to 500 ml) water

Lunch
- Julienne Salad: 1 hard-boiled egg, 1 oz (30 g) sliced ham, and 1 oz (30 g) part-skim cheese served on 1 to 2 cups (250 to 500 ml) mixed greens with 4 tsp low-fat (20 ml) dressing
- 1 small whole-grain roll (3 oz/90 g serving)
- 1 to 2 cups (250 to 500 ml) water

Afternoon snack
- 1 sliced medium apple with 1 tbsp (15 ml) almond butter
- 1 to 2 cups (250 to 500 ml) water

Dinner
- Herbed Pork Tenderloin (p. 306)
- 1/2 cup (125 ml) baby new potatoes, roasted
- 1 to 2 cups (250 to 500 ml) mixed greens with 4 tsp (20 ml) low-fat dressing
- 1 to 2 cups (250 to 500 ml) water

Leslie's tip: The recipe for Herbed Pork Tenderloin serves four people. If you're cooking for one or two people, save the leftover pork for tomorrow's lunch—Pork Souvlaki. If you plan to use all the pork tonight, cook an extra tenderloin to use for Thursday's lunch.

Nutrient breakdown: 1351 cal, 77 g pro, 43 g total fat (8 g sat. fat), 176 g carb, 25 g fibre, 295 mg chol, 2009 mg sodium

Week 5: Thursday

Breakfast
* 1 cup (250 ml) mixed fresh fruit sprinkled with 1/3 cup (75 ml) Cranberry Apple Granola (p. 283)
* 12 oz (350 ml) latte, made with skim or 1% milk, or calcium-enriched soy milk OR 1 Milk and Milk Alternative serving of your choice
* Coffee, tea, or water

Morning snack
* Strawberry Sunrise Smoothie (p. 289)

Lunch
* Pork Souvlaki: Stuff one-half 6 inch (15 cm) whole-wheat pita pocket with 2 oz (60 g) cooked pork tenderloin, chopped tomato, and cucumber; top with 2 tbsp (25 ml) tzatziki
* 1 to 2 cups (250 to 500 ml) mixed greens with lemon juice or seasoned rice vinegar as dressing
* 1 to 2 cups (250 to 500 ml) water

Afternoon snack
* 1 cup (250 ml) mixed raw veggie sticks with 2 tbsp (25 ml) hummus
* 1 to 2 cups (250 to 500 ml) water

Dinner
* Tomato Herb Pasta with Veggie Ground Round (p. 325)
* 1 to 2 cups (250 to 500 ml) mixed greens with 4 tsp (20 ml) low-fat dressing
* 1 to 2 cups (250 to 500 ml) water

Leslie's tip: If you don't like soy, replace the ground round with 1 pound (454 g) extra-lean ground beef, chicken, or turkey.

Nutrient breakdown: 1402 cal, 85 g pro, 28 g total fat (6 g sat. fat), 221 g carb, 37 g fibre, 76 mg chol, 1662 mg sodium

Week 5: Friday

Breakfast

- 1 poached egg on 1 slice whole-grain toast
- 1/4 medium cantaloupe, sliced
- Coffee, tea, or water

Leslie's tip: Save the leftover melon for Saturday morning's fruit salad recipe.

Morning snack

- 3/4 cup (175 ml or 175 g container) low-fat (1% MF or less) plain or flavoured yogurt
- 1 to 2 cups (250 to 500 ml) water

Lunch

- Turkey Sandwich: 2 oz (60 g) sliced turkey breast with Dijon mustard, sliced tomato, and romaine lettuce on 2 slices whole-grain rye bread
- 1 cup (250 ml) vegetable soup, homemade or commercial brand with less than 600 milligrams sodium per serving
- 1 to 2 cups (250 to 500 ml) water

Afternoon snack

- 6 walnut halves
- 1/4 cup (50 ml) dried fruit
- 1 to 2 cups (250 to 500 ml) water

Dinner

- Salmon Burger (p. 297) in a 6 inch (15 cm) whole-wheat pita
- 1 to 2 cups (250 to 500 ml) Spinach Salad: Combine baby spinach leaves with sliced tomatoes, red onion, and mushrooms; top with 4 tsp (20 ml) Poppy Seed Dressing (p. 333)
- 1 to 2 cups (250 to 500 ml) water

Nutrient breakdown: 1376 cal, 89 g pro, 37 g total fat (8 g sat. fat), 182 g carb, 22 g fibre, 351 mg chol, 2125 mg sodium

Week 5: Saturday

Breakfast

- 1/2 to 3/4 cup (125 to 175 ml) whole-grain cereal topped with 3/4 cup (175 ml or 175 g container) low-fat (1% MF or less) plain or flavoured yogurt and 1 tbsp (15 ml) sunflower seeds
- 1 cup (250 ml) Fresh Fruit Salad (p. 287)
- Coffee, tea, or water

Lunch

- 2 cups (500 ml) Hearty Black Bean Soup (p. 292) OR Red Pepper Lentil Soup (p. 292) OR minestrone
- 1 small whole-grain roll (3 oz/90 g serving) OR 1 Starchy Food serving of your choice
- 1 to 2 cups (250 to 500 ml) water

Afternoon snack

- Cranberry Swirl Smoothie (p. 287)

Dinner

- 2 Chicken Fajitas (p. 303)
- 2 cups (500 ml) mixed greens with 4 tsp (20 ml) low-fat dressing
- 1 to 2 cups (250 to 500 ml) water

Nutrient breakdown: 1504 cal, 76 g pro, 27 g total fat (4 g sat. fat), 263 g carb, 46 g fibre, 57 mg chol, 1522 mg sodium

Week 5: Sunday

Breakfast

- Breakfast Egg Sandwich: Fry 1 egg in a non-stick pan, then place on a toasted whole-wheat English muffin with 1 oz (30 g) lean smoked ham; add sliced tomato
- 1/2 cup (125 ml) unsweetened fruit juice
- Coffee, tea, or water

Lunch

- Open-Faced Tuna Melt: Mix 2 oz (60 g) water-packed light tuna with 2 tsp (10 ml) low-fat mayonnaise and spices as desired. Top 2 slices toasted whole-grain bread with tuna salad and 1 oz grated part-skim cheddar cheese; broil until cheese is melted and bubbly
- 1 cup (250 ml) mixed greens with 2 tsp (10 ml) low-fat dressing
- 1 cup (250 ml) skim or 1% milk, or calcium-enriched plain soy milk

Afternoon snack

- 3/4 cup (175 ml or 175 g container) low-fat (1% MF or less) plain or flavoured yogurt topped with 1/2 cup (125 ml) blueberries and 2 tbsp (25 ml) slivered almonds
- 1 to 2 cups (250 to 500 ml) water

Leslie's tip: If fresh blueberries are not in season, buy them frozen. Defrost in the microwave, then add to yogurt. Alternatively, add 2 tablespoons (25 ml) dried blueberries to your snack.

Dinner

- 1 1/2 cups (375 ml) Whole-Grain Lentil Casserole (p. 328)
- 1 cup (250 ml) steamed broccoli florets and carrots
- 1 to 2 cups (250 to 500 ml) water

Nutrient breakdown: 1339 cal, 83 g pro, 30 g total fat (6 g sat. fat), 194 g carb, 29 g fibre, 235 mg chol, 2411 mg sodium

Week 6: Monday

Breakfast

- 1/2 cup (125 ml) cooked oatmeal or 1 package instant unflavoured oatmeal, topped with 1/2 cup (125 ml) blueberries and 1 tbsp (15 ml) chopped walnuts
- 12 oz (350 ml) latte, made with skim or 1% milk, or calcium-enriched soy milk OR 1 Milk and Milk Alternative serving of your choice
- Coffee, tea, or water

Leslie's tip: All types of cooked oatmeal—steel cut, long cooking, quick cooking, one-minute, and instant—deliver 4 grams of fibre per 1/2 cup (125 ml) serving. But only steel cut and long-cooking oats have a low glycemic index. That means they are digested slowly and converted gradually to blood sugar, helping you feel full and energized longer after your meal.

Morning snack

- 1 fruit serving of your choice
- 1 oz (30 g) part-skim cheese or 1 part-skim cheese string
- 1 to 2 cups (250 to 500 ml) water

Lunch

- Turkey Wrap: Place 3 oz (90 g) roasted turkey breast in a 10 inch (25 cm) whole-wheat tortilla with 2 tbsp (25 ml) hummus, lettuce leaves, sliced tomato, shredded carrots, and sliced red onion
- 1 to 2 cups (250 to 500 ml) water

Afternoon snack

- 3/4 cup (175 ml or 175 g container) low-fat (1% MF or less) plain or flavoured yogurt
- 1 fruit serving of your choice
- 1 to 2 cups (250 to 500 ml) water

Dinner

- Cajun Fish (p. 293)
- 2/3 cup (150 ml) steamed wild rice
- 1/2 cup (125 ml) steamed green beans
- Baked Tomato: Remove the core of 1 tomato, sprinkle with dried basil and grated Parmesan cheese, and bake at 350°F (180°C) for 15 to 20 minutes
- 1 to 2 cups (250 to 500 ml) water

Nutrient breakdown: 1342 cal, 92 g pro, 26 g total fat (5 g sat. fat), 192 g carb, 23 g fibre, 104 mg chol, 937 mg sodium

Week 6: Tuesday

Breakfast

- 3/4 to 1 cup (175 to 250 ml) whole-grain cereal, topped with 2 tbsp (25 ml) ground flaxseed and 1 medium peach, sliced
- 1 cup (250 ml) skim or 1% milk, or calcium-enriched plain soy milk
- Coffee, tea, water

Morning snack

- 3/4 cup (175 ml or 175 g container) low-fat (1% MF or less) plain or flavoured yogurt
- 1 to 2 cups (250 to 500 ml) water

Lunch

- Lentil Soup with Turkey Sausage (p. 291)
- 1 to 2 cups (250 to 500 ml) mixed greens with 4 tsp (20 ml) low-fat dressing
- 1 to 2 cups (250 to 500 ml) water

Afternoon snack

- 1/2 to 1 cup (125 to 250 ml) veggie sticks with 2 tbsp (25 ml) hummus
- 1 to 2 cups (250 to 500 ml) water

Dinner

- Chicken Mango Stir-Fry (p. 304)
- 2/3 cup (150 ml) steamed basmati rice
- 1 to 2 cups (250 to 500 ml) water

Leslie's tip: Cook extra chicken breast for tomorrow's lunch—Grilled Chicken Salad.

Nutrient breakdown: 1339 cal, 82 g pro, 26 g total fat (4 g sat. fat), 224 g carb, 47 g fibre, 65 mg chol, 2288 mg sodium

Week 6: Wednesday

Breakfast
* Peachy Delight Smoothie (p. 288)
* 1 slice whole-grain toast with sugar-reduced fruit spread

Morning snack
* 12 oz (350 ml) latte, made with skim or 1% milk, or calcium-enriched soy milk, OR 1 Milk and Milk Alternative serving of your choice
* 1 fruit serving of your choice
* 1 to 2 cups (250 to 500 ml) water

Lunch
* Grilled Chicken Salad: Top 2 cups (500 ml) mixed greens with 2 oz (60 g) grilled chicken breast, 1 oz (30 g) goat cheese, 1 tbsp (15 ml) toasted pine nuts, 2 tbsp (25 ml) chopped sun-dried tomatoes, and 4 tsp (20 ml) low-fat dressing
* 100% whole-grain crispbread crackers (3 Wasa or 6 Ryvita)
* 1 to 2 cups (250 to 500 ml) water

Afternoon snack
* 3 cups (750 ml) plain air-popped or microwave light popcorn
* 1 to 2 cups (250 to 500 ml) water

Dinner
* Veggie Burger: Place 1 soy-based veggie burger in a 6 inch (15 cm) whole-wheat pita, add lettuce leaves, sliced tomato, sliced onion, mustard, and relish if desired
* 1 to 2 cups (250 to 500 ml) mixed greens with 4 tsp (20 ml) low-fat dressing
* 1 to 2 cups (250 to 500 ml) water

Leslie's tip: Most veggie burgers are lower in calories, fat, and saturated fat than a beef burger—and they're higher in fibre. When shopping for soy-based patties, read the labels. Choose a brand that has no more than 4 grams of fat and 1 gram of saturated fat, zero grams of trans fat, and no more than 400 milligrams of sodium per patty. My favourites include Yves veggie burgers, Amy's Texas Burger, and Sole Cuisine's veggie burgers.

Nutrient breakdown: 1361 cal, 88 g pro, 36 g total fat (15 g sat. fat), 181 g carb, 32 g fibre, 102 mg chol, 2076 mg sodium

Week 6: Thursday

Breakfast
- 1 boiled egg
- 1 slice whole-grain toast
- 1/2 cup (125 ml) unsweetened fruit juice OR 1 Fruit serving of your choice
- Coffee, tea, or water

Morning snack
- Very Berry Smoothie (p. 289)

Lunch
- Roast Beef Sandwich: 3 oz (90 g) sliced lean roast beef, lettuce, sliced tomato, sliced red onion, mustard or horseradish on 2 slices whole-grain rye bread
- 1 to 2 cups (250 to 500 ml) water

Afternoon snack
- 3/4 cup (175 ml or 175 g container) low-fat (1% MF or less) plain or flavoured yogurt
- 1 fruit serving of your choice
- 1 to 2 cups (250 to 500 ml) water

Dinner
- Citrus Mustard Trout (p. 293)
- 1 cup (250 ml) Pepper and Snow Pea Sauté (p. 330)
- 4 roasted or boiled baby new potatoes
- 1 to 2 cups (250 to 500 ml) water

Leslie's tip: If you can't find trout at your fish market, consider buying frozen. These days, you can find many types of unbreaded frozen fish fillets at the grocery store—including trout. They're convenient and just as nutritious as their fresh counterparts.

Nutrient breakdown: 1420 cal, 88 g pro, 27 g total fat (8 g sat. fat), 214 g carb, 23 g fibre, 332 mg chol, 1095 mg sodium

Week 6: Friday

Breakfast
- 3/4 to 1 cup (175 to 250 ml) whole-grain cereal topped with 1 tbsp (15 ml) ground flaxseed, 1/2 sliced banana, and 1/2 cup (125 ml) blueberries
- 1 cup (250 ml) skim or 1% milk, or calcium-enriched plain soy milk

Morning snack
- 1 cup (250 ml) veggie sticks with 2 tbsp (25 ml) hummus
- 1 to 2 cups (250 to 500 ml) water

Lunch
- 1 1/2 cups (375 ml) black bean or lentil soup (homemade or store bought)
- 7 whole-wheat soda crackers
- 1/2 cup (125 ml) bell pepper strips
- 1 to 2 cups (250 to 500 ml) water

Afternoon snack
- 1 fruit serving of your choice
- 1 oz (30 g) part-skim cheese
- 1 to 2 cups (250 to 500 ml) water

Dinner
- Indian Yogurt Chicken (p. 308)
- 2/3 cup (150 ml) steamed basmati rice
- 1/2 cup (125 ml) each steamed spinach and carrots
- 1 to 2 cups (250 to 500 ml) water

Leslie's tip: For extra flavour and texture, garnish the chicken with chopped cilantro and chopped pecans. Serve with your favourite homemade or store-bought chutney.

Nutrient breakdown: 1395 cal, 68 g pro, 26 g total fat (5 g sat. fat), 250 g carb, 50 g fibre, 64 mg chol, 1522 mg sodium

Week 6: Saturday

Breakfast
- 2 slices whole-grain toast with 1 1/2 tsp (7 ml) peanut butter and 1/2 sliced banana
- 12 oz (350 ml) latte, made with skim or 1% milk, or calcium-enriched soy milk, OR 1 Milk and Milk Alternative serving of your choice
- Coffee, tea, or water

Lunch
- Mediterranean Tuna Salad: Top 1 to 2 cups (250 to 500 ml) mixed greens with 3 oz (90 g) water-packed light tuna, 2 tbsp (25 ml) raisins, 6 medium olives (green or black), 1/3 cup (75 ml) chickpeas, shredded carrot, halved cherry tomatoes, and 4 tsp (20 ml) low-fat dressing
- 1 fruit serving of your choice
- 1 to 2 cups (250 to 500 ml) water

Afternoon snack
- 3 Whole-Wheat Pita Chips (p. 285) with White Bean Dip (p. 327)
- 1 to 2 cups (250 to 500 ml) water

Dinner
- 4 oz (120 g) Teriyaki Sirloin Steak (p. 313)
- 1/2 baked potato topped with 2 tbsp (25 ml) low-fat plain yogurt mixed with 2 tbsp (25 ml) low-fat salsa
- 1 cup (250 ml) grilled red bell peppers and zucchini
- 1 to 2 cups (250 to 500 ml) water

Nutrient breakdown: 1417 cal, 92 g pro, 31 g total fat (7 g sat. fat), 204 g carb, 23 g fibre, 102 mg chol, 1605 mg sodium

Week 6: Sunday

Breakfast

- Breakfast Omelet (p. 286)
- 1 slice whole-grain toast with 1 1/2 tsp (7 ml) nut butter
- 12 oz (350 ml) latte made with skim or soy milk OR 1 Milk and Milk Alternative serving of your choice
- Coffee, tea, or water

Lunch

- Open-Faced Salmon Sandwich: Mix 2 oz (60 g) canned salmon with 2 tbsp (25 ml) low-fat mayonnaise, 1 tsp (5 ml) chopped fresh dill, and 1/4 cup (50 ml) chopped celery; place on 1 slice whole-grain bread
- 1 cup (250 ml) Fresh Fruit Salad (p. 287)
- 1 to 2 cups (250 to 500 ml) water

Afternoon snack

- Peachy Delight Smoothie (p. 288)

Dinner

- 1 slice Turkey Lasagna (p. 318)
- 2 cups (500 ml) romaine lettuce with 4 tsp (20 ml) low-fat Caesar dressing
- 1 to 2 cups (250 to 500 ml) water

Leslie's tip: The recipe for Turkey Lasagna serves nine people. To practice portion control, make sure you divide the dish into nine pieces before taking a serving.

Nutrient breakdown: 1465 cal, 99 g pro, 44 g total fat (13 g sat. fat), 177 g carb, 21 g fibre, 468 mg chol, 2339 mg sodium

Week 7: Monday

Breakfast

- 1 breakfast-sized whole-grain pita with 2 tsp (10 ml) reduced-sugar fruit spread and 1 1/2 tsp (7 ml) nut butter
- 3/4 cup (175 ml or 175 g container) low-fat (1% MF or less) plain or flavoured yogurt with 1 cup (250 ml) mixed berries
- Coffee, tea, or water

Morning snack

- 1/4 cup (50 ml) 1% MF or fat-free cottage cheese with 1/2 cup (125 ml) pineapple chunks or fruit salad
- 1 to 2 cups (250 to 500 ml) water

Lunch

- Greek Wrap: Place 2 oz (60 g) roasted pork tenderloin and 1 oz (30 g) part-skim feta cheese in a 10 inch (25 cm) soft whole-grain tortilla with lettuce, tomato leaves, sliced onion, sliced cucumber, and 2 tbsp (25 ml) tzatziki
- 1 to 2 cups (250 to 500 ml) water

Afternoon snack

- 1/2 to 1 cup (125 to 250 ml) raw vegetables with 2 tbsp (25 ml) low-fat ranch dip
- 1 to 2 cups (250 to 500 ml) water

Dinner

- 3 oz (90 g) grilled turkey breast
- 2/3 cup (150 ml) Steamed Quinoa (p. 284)
- 1 to 2 cups (250 to 500 ml) mixed greens with sliced vegetables and 4 tsp (20 ml) low-fat dressing
- 1 to 2 cups (250 to 500 ml) water

Nutrient breakdown: 1330 cal, 88 g pro, 28 g total fat (6 g sat. fat), 188 g carb, 20 g fibre, 139 mg chol, 1982 mg sodium

Week 7: Tuesday

Breakfast
- 1/2 cup (125 ml) hot oat bran cereal, topped with 2 tbsp (25 ml) ground flaxseed and 2 tbsp (25 ml) raisins
- 12 oz (350 ml) latte, made with skim or 1% milk, or calcium-enriched soy milk OR 1 Milk and Milk Alternative serving of your choice
- Coffee, tea, or water

Morning snack
- Mango Tango Smoothie (p. 288)

Lunch
- Chicken Salad Sandwich: Mix 3 oz (90 g) cooked, shredded chicken with 4 tsp (20 ml) low-fat mayonnaise and spices as desired; serve on 1 small whole-grain roll with sliced tomatoes
- 2 cups (500 ml) Spinach Salad: Combine baby spinach leaves with sliced red onion, mushrooms, and shredded carrot; top with 4 tsp (20 ml) low-fat salad dressing
- 1 to 2 cups (250 to 500 ml) water

Afternoon snack
- 1 low-fat granola bar
- 1 to 2 cups (250 to 500 ml) water

Leslie's tip: Read labels when buying granola bars. Choose one that has at least 2 grams of fibre, zero grams of trans fat, and no more than 1 gram of saturated fat and 10 grams of sugar per serving.

Dinner
- 3 oz (90 g) Maple Glazed Salmon (p. 296)
- 2/3 cup (150 ml) steamed brown rice
- 1/2 cup (125 ml) each steamed snow peas and carrots
- 1 to 2 cups (250 to 500 ml) water

Nutrient breakdown: 1462 cal, 86 g pro, 39 g total fat (8 g sat. fat), 213 g carb, 34 g fibre, 146 mg chol, 1762 mg sodium

Week 7: Wednesday

Breakfast

- 1/3 cup (75 ml) Cranberry Apple Granola (p. 285) with 3/4 cup (175 ml or 175 g container) low-fat (1% MF or less) plain or flavoured yogurt, topped with 1/2 sliced banana and 1/2 cup (125 ml) blueberries
- Coffee, tea, or water

Morning snack

- 12 oz (350 ml) latte, made with skim or 1% milk, or calcium-enriched soy milk OR 1 Milk and Milk Alternative serving of your choice

Lunch

- 1 1/2 cups (375 ml) Hearty Black Bean Soup (p. 290)
- 1 to 2 cups (250 to 500 ml) mixed greens with 4 tsp (20 ml) low-fat dressing
- 1 to 2 cups (250 to 500 ml) water

Afternoon snack

- 1 medium orange with 10 plain, unsalted almonds
- 1 to 2 cups (250 to 500 ml) water

Dinner

- 1 Turkey Burrito (p. 316)
- 1 to 2 cups (250 to 500 ml) mixed greens with lemon juice or seasoned rice vinegar as dressing
- 1 to 2 cups (250 to 500 ml) water

Nutrient breakdown: 1424 cal, 75 g pro, 32 g total fat (7 g sat. fat), 218 g carb, 33 g fibre, 77 mg chol, 1885 mg sodium

Week 7: Thursday

Breakfast
- 1 slice whole-grain toast with 1 1/2 tsp (7 ml) nut butter
- 1 small banana OR 1 Fruit serving of your choice
- Coffee, tea, or water

Morning snack
- Very Berry Smoothie (p. 289)

Lunch
- Open-Faced Ham and Cheese Sandwich: 2 oz (60 g) ham with 1 oz (30 g) part-skim cheese with 1 tbsp (15 ml) low-fat mayonnaise, Dijon mustard, lettuce, and sliced tomato on 1 slice whole-grain toast
- 1 to 2 cups (250 to 500 ml) water

Afternoon snack
- 1/2 whole-wheat pita and 2 tbsp (25 ml) hummus
- 1 to 2 cups (250 to 500 ml) water

Dinner
- Sweet and Sour Tofu Stir-Fry (p. 323)
- 1 cup (250 ml) cooked rice noodles
- 1 cup (250 ml) steamed greens (e.g., Swiss chard, spinach, rapini, kale); drizzle with 1 tsp (5 ml) sesame oil, then sprinkle 1/2 tsp (2 ml) toasted sesame seeds overtop
- 1 to 2 cups (250 to 500 ml) water

Nutrient breakdown: 1502 cal, 70 g pro, 41 g total fat (6 g sat. fat), 235 g carb, 31 g fibre, 42 mg chol, 2406 mg sodium

Week 7: Friday

Breakfast

- 1 cup (250 ml) whole-grain cereal, topped with 1 tbsp (15 ml) ground flaxseed
- 1 cup (250 ml) skim or 1% milk, or calcium-enriched plain soy milk
- 1/2 cup (125 ml) unsweetened fruit juice
- Coffee, tea, or water

Morning snack

- 3/4 cup (175 ml or 175 g container) low-fat (1% MF or less) plain or flavoured yogurt with 1 cup (250 ml) mixed berries and 1 tbsp (15 ml) sunflower seeds
- 1 to 2 cups (250 to 500 ml) water

Lunch

- Tuna Salad: Place 3 oz (90 g) water-packed light tuna on 2 cups (500 ml) mixed greens; add 3 tbsp (50 ml) dried cranberries, shredded carrot, sliced cucumber, sliced tomato, and 1 oz (30 g) crumbled feta cheese; dress with 4 tsp (20 ml) low-fat dressing
- 1 to 2 cups (250 to 500 ml) water

Afternoon snack

- 1 cup (250 ml) baby carrots with 2 tbsp (25 ml) low-fat dip
- 1 to 2 cups (250 to 500 ml) water

Dinner

- 3 oz (90 g) Orange Rosemary Chicken (p. 309)
- 2/3 cup (150 ml) steamed wild or brown rice
- 1 cup (250 ml) Brussels sprouts roasted with 2 tsp (10 ml) canola oil
- 1 to 2 cups (250 to 500 ml) water

Leslie's tip: Brussels sprouts are delicious roasted. To roast, cut them in half lengthwise and place them cut side up on a baking sheet or in a shallow roasting pan. Drizzle with canola oil and sprinkle with salt and pepper. Roast at 400°F (200°C) for 25 to 30 minutes.

Nutrient breakdown: 1296 cal, 99 g pro, 24 g total fat (4 g sat. fat), 202 g carb, 53 g fibre, 90 mg chol, 1489 mg sodium

Week 7: Saturday

Breakfast

- 1 poached egg
- 1 slice whole-grain toast with 1 1/2 tsp (7 ml) nut butter
- Cranberry Swirl Smoothie (p. 287)
- Coffee, tea, or water

Lunch

- 1 cup (250 ml) Mexican Bean Salad (p. 320)
- Whole-grain crispbread crackers (e.g., 1 1/2 Wasa or 3 Ryvita) or 1/2 whole-wheat pita pocket
- 1/2 to 1 cup (125 to 250 ml) veggie sticks with 2 tbsp (25 ml) low-fat ranch dip
- 1 to 2 cups (250 to 500 ml) water

Afternoon snack

- 3 cups (750 ml) of plain air-popped or light microwave popcorn
- 1 to 2 cups (250 to 500 ml) water

Dinner

- 4 oz (120 g) Sesame Soy Trout (p. 298)
- 1/2 medium baked potato with 1/4 cup (50 ml) fat-free sour cream
- 1/2 cup (125 ml) broccoli and 1/2 cup (125 ml) red bell pepper strips sautéed in 2 tsp (10 ml) canola oil
- 1 to 2 cups (250 to 500 ml) water

Nutrient breakdown: 1394 cal, 76 g pro, 36 g total fat (9 g sat. fat), 207 g carb, 38 g fibre, 278 mg chol, 913 mg sodium

Week 7: Sunday

Breakfast

- 2 slices French Toast (p. 286) with 2 tsp (10 ml) reduced-sugar fruit spread and 1 1/2 tsp (7 ml) nut butter
- 1 cup (250 ml) Fresh Fruit Salad (p. 287)
- 12 oz (350 ml) latte, made with skim or 1% milk, or calcium-enriched soy milk OR 1 Milk and Milk Alternative serving of your choice
- Coffee, tea, or water

Lunch

- Open-Faced Salmon Sandwich: 2 oz (60 g) canned salmon, 1 tbsp (15 ml) low-fat mayonnaise, lettuce, sliced tomato, sliced onion, and salt and pepper to taste, on 1 slice whole-grain bread
- 1 to 2 cups (250 to 500 ml) mixed greens with 4 tsp (20 ml) low-fat dressing
- 1 to 2 cups (250 to 500 ml) water

Afternoon snack

- Strawberry Sunrise Smoothie (p. 289)

Dinner

- 4 oz (120 g) Honey Mustard Chicken (p. 307)
- 1/3 cup (75 ml) steamed brown rice
- 1 cup (250 ml) vegetables (e.g., red bell pepper strips, broccoli, carrots) sautéed in 2 tsp (10 ml) canola oil
- 1 to 2 cups (250 to 500 ml) water

Nutrient breakdown: 1326 cal, 74 g pro, 39 g total fat (9 g sat. fat), 183 g carb, 22 g fibre, 273 mg chol, 1403 mg sodium

Week 8: Monday

Breakfast
* 1/2 cup (125 ml) cooked oatmeal or 1 package instant unflavoured oatmeal with 2 tbsp (25 ml) raisins
* 3/4 cup (175 ml or 175 g container) low-fat vanilla yogurt
* Coffee, tea, or water

Morning snack
* 12 oz (350 ml) latte, made with skim or 1% milk, or calcium-enriched soy milk OR 1 Milk and Milk Alternative serving of your choice
* 1 fruit serving of your choice

Lunch
* Salmon Pasta Salad (p. 292)
* 1 to 2 cups (250 to 500 ml) water

Afternoon snack
* 1 medium pear with 6 walnut halves
* 1 to 2 cups (250 to 500 ml) water

Dinner
* 1 Chickpea Burger (p. 319) served on 1 small whole-grain roll
* 1 to 2 cups (250 to 500 ml) mixed greens with 4 tsp (20 ml) low-fat dressing
* 1 to 2 cups (250 to 500 ml) water

Nutrient breakdown: 1354 cal, 70 g pro, 43 g total fat (7 g sat. fat), 186 g carb, 22 g fibre, 90 mg chol, 1168 mg sodium

Week 8: Tuesday

Breakfast

- 1 slice whole-grain toast with 1 1/2 tsp (7 ml) nut butter
- Peachy Delight Smoothie (p. 288)
- Coffee, tea, or water

Morning snack

- 1 fruit serving of your choice with 1 oz (30 g) part-skim cheese
- 1 to 2 cups (250 to 500 ml) water

Lunch

- Open-Faced Ham Sandwich: 3 oz (90 g) ham, 1 tbsp (15 ml) low-fat mayonnaise, spinach leaves, and sliced tomato on 1 slice whole-grain rye bread
- 1 to 2 cups (250 to 500 ml) cups mixed greens with 4 tsp (20 ml) low-fat dressing
- 1 cup (250 ml) skim or 1% milk, or calcium-enriched plain soy milk

Afternoon snack

- 2 oz (60 g) mini-can seasoned tuna with 7 whole-wheat soda crackers
- 1 to 2 cups (250 to 500 ml) water

Dinner

- 3 oz (90 g) Honey Garlic Chicken (p. 306)
- 2/3 cup (150 ml) steamed basmati rice
- 1 cup (250 ml) Balsamic Roasted Asparagus (p. 329)
- 1 to 2 cups (250 to 500 ml) water

Nutrient breakdown: 1346 cal, 92 g pro, 32 g total fat (9 g sat. fat), 182 g carb, 21 g fibre, 136 mg chol, 2697 mg sodium

Week 8: Wednesday

Breakfast

- 1/2 to 3/4 cup (125 to 175 ml) whole-grain cereal, topped with 1 tbsp (15 ml) ground flaxseed
- 1 cup (250 ml) mixed berries
- 1 cup (250 ml) skim or 1% milk, or calcium-enriched plain soy milk
- Coffee, tea, or water

Morning snack

- 3/4 cup (175 ml or 175 g container) low-fat (1% MF or less) plain or flavoured yogurt
- 1 to 2 cups (250 to 500 ml) water

Lunch

- 1 1/2 cups (375 ml) Hearty Black Bean Soup (p. 290)
- 7 whole-grain soda crackers OR 1 Starchy Food serving of your choice
- 1 to 2 cups (250 to 500 ml) cups mixed greens with 4 tsp (20 ml) low-fat dressing
- 1 to 2 cups (250 to 500 ml) water

Afternoon snack

- 1 cup (250 ml) assorted veggie sticks with 2 tbsp (25 ml) low-fat ranch dip
- 1 to 2 cups (250 to 500 ml) water

Dinner

- Cumin Citrus Pork (p. 305)
- 1 small baked potato topped with 2 tbsp (25 ml) fat-free sour cream
- 1 cup (250 ml) vegetables (e.g., red bell pepper strips, broccoli, carrots) sautéed in 2 tsp (10 ml) canola oil
- 1 to 2 cups (250 to 500 ml) water

Nutrient breakdown: 1354 cal, 79 g pro, 24 g total fat (7 g sat. fat), 232 g carb, 48 g fibre, 78 mg chol, 2393 mg sodium

Week 8: Thursday

Breakfast
- 1 poached egg with 2 slices whole-grain toast and 1 1/2 tsp (7 ml) nut butter
- 1/2 cup (125 ml) unsweetened fruit juice
- Coffee, tea, or water

Morning snack
- 1 Fruit serving of your choice with 1 oz (30 g) part-skim cheese
- 1 to 2 cups (250 to 500 ml) water

Lunch
- Chicken Wrap: Place 3 oz (90 g) roasted chicken breast in a 10 inch (25 cm) soft whole-wheat tortilla; add lettuce or spinach leaves, sliced tomato, and sliced onion; drizzle with 4 tsp (20 ml) low-fat dressing; wrap up and enjoy
- 1 1/2 cups (375 ml) vegetable soup
- 1 to 2 cups (250 to 500 ml) water

Afternoon snack
- 3/4 cup (175 ml or 175 g container) low-fat (1% MF or less) plain or flavoured yogurt topped with 2 tbsp (25 ml) low-fat granola
- 1 to 2 cups (250 to 500 ml) water

Dinner
- 4 oz (120 g) Sole with Gremolata Sauce (p. 299)
- 1/3 (75 ml) cup steamed wild or brown rice
- 1 cup (250 ml) steamed spinach
- 1/2 cup (125 ml) steamed carrots
- 1 to 2 cups (250 to 500 ml) water

Nutrient breakdown: 1417 cal, 97 g pro, 29 g total fat (6 g sat. fat), 196 g carb, 25 g fibre, 332 mg chol, 2929 mg sodium

Week 8: Friday

Breakfast
- 1 breakfast-sized pita with 1 1/2 tsp (7 ml) nut butter and 2 tsp (10 ml) sugar-reduced fruit spread
- 1 fruit serving of your choice
- Coffee, tea, or water

Morning snack
- Friendly Flax Smoothie (p. 288)

Lunch
- Tuna on Mixed Greens: Top 2 cups (500 ml) mixed greens with 2 oz (60 g) water-packed light tuna and 1 oz (30 g) cheddar cheese; add chopped vegetables as desired; dress with 4 tsp (20 ml) low-fat dressing
- 1 to 2 cups (250 to 500 ml) water

Afternoon snack
- 3/4 cup (175 ml or 175 g container) low-fat (1% MF or less) plain or flavoured yogurt with 1/2 cup (125 ml) mixed berries
- 1 to 2 cups (250 to 500 ml) water

Dinner
- 2 Chicken Fajitas (p. 303)
- 1 cup (250 ml) mixed greens with lemon juice or seasoned rice vinegar as dressing
- 1 to 2 cups (250 to 500 ml) water

Nutrient breakdown: 1327 cal, 82 g pro, 34 g total fat (11 g sat. fat), 186 g carb, 24 g fibre, 110 mg chol, 1535 mg sodium

Week 8: Saturday

Breakfast
- 1 slice whole-grain toast with 1 1/2 tsp (7 ml) nut butter
- 1 small banana
- 12 oz (350 ml) latte, made with skim or 1% milk, or calcium-enriched soy milk OR 1 Milk and Milk Alternative serving of your choice
- Coffee, tea, or water

Lunch
- Salmon Sandwich: 3 oz (90 g) canned salmon mixed with 2 tbsp (25 ml) low-fat mayonnaise, salt, and pepper, with lettuce leaves, sliced tomato, and sliced cucumber on 2 slices whole-grain bread
- 1 to 2 cups (250 to 500 ml) water

Afternoon snack
- 3/4 cup (175 ml or 175 g container) low-fat (1% MF or less) plain or flavoured yogurt
- 1 to 2 cups (250 to 500 ml) water

Dinner
- Vegetarian Chili (p. 326)
- 1/2 medium baked potato, topped with 3 tbsp (50 ml) fat-free sour cream
- 2 cups (500 ml) mixed greens with 4 tsp (20 ml) low-fat dressing
- 1 to 2 cups (250 to 500 ml) water

Nutrient breakdown: 1384 cal, 84 g pro, 36 g total fat (10 g sat. fat), 193 g carb, 29 g fibre, 67 mg chol, 1873 mg sodium

Week 8: Sunday

Breakfast

- 1 boiled or poached egg
- 1 slice whole-grain toast with 2 tsp (10 ml) reduced-sugar fruit spread
- 1/2 cup (125 ml) unsweetened fruit juice
- Coffee, tea, or water

Lunch

- 1 cup (250 ml) Vegetarian Chili (p. 326) with 1 oz (30 g) grated part-skim cheese
- 1/2 whole-grain pita pocket
- 1 to 2 cups (250 to 500 ml) Spinach Salad: Combine baby spinach leaves with sliced tomato, red onion, mushrooms, and shredded carrot; top with 4 tsp (20 ml) low-fat dressing
- 1 to 2 cups (250 to 500 ml) water

Afternoon snack

- Very Berry Smoothie (p. 289)

Dinner

- Roasted Chicken Breast with Vegetables and New Potatoes: 4 oz (120 g) chicken breast, 4 small new potatoes, 1/2 cup (125 ml) sliced carrots, 1/2 cup (125 ml) chopped celery, 2 tsp (10 ml) canola oil. Preheat oven to 375°F (190°C). Lightly coat chicken breast with non-stick cooking spray and place in a glass baking dish. Cut potatoes, carrots, and celery into 1 inch (2.5 cm) pieces, lightly coat with canola oil, and place in dish with chicken. Season with salt, pepper, dried thyme, and dried rosemary. Cover and roast for 45 to 50 minutes or until potatoes are tender and chicken is cooked through.
- 1 to 2 cups (250 to 500 ml) water

Nutrient breakdown: 1423 cal, 86 g pro, 28 g total fat (5 g sat. fat), 220 g carb, 37 g fibre, 304 mg chol, 1508 mg sodium

7

The No-Fail Diet Recipes

Contents

Cereals and Grains

Cranberry Apple Granola

4 cups	large-flake oats	1 L
1/4 cup	slivered almonds	50 ml
1/4 cup	sunflower seeds	50 ml
1/2 cup	unsweetened applesauce	125 ml
1/3 cup	honey	75 ml
2 tsp	cinnamon	10 ml
2 tsp	canola oil	10 ml
1/2 tsp	ground ginger	2 ml
1 cup	dried apples, chopped	250 ml
1/2 cup	dried cranberries	125 ml

Preheat oven to 375°F (190°C).

In a large bowl, combine oats, almonds, and sunflower seeds.

Combine applesauce, honey, cinnamon, oil, and ginger. Pour over oat mixture and mix well, until coated evenly.

Spread mixture on a jelly-roll pan and bake for 20 minutes. Gently stir granola; bake an additional 5 to 10 minutes or until dry.

Cool; stir in apples and cranberries.

Store in an airtight container.

1 serving equals 1/3 cup (75 ml).

Makes 18 servings (6 cups/1.5 L)

Per serving: 201 cal, 7 g pro, 5 g total fat (1 g sat. fat), 34 g carb, 5 g fibre, 0 mg chol, 6 mg sodium

Leslie's Overnight Muesli

2 cups	steel-cut oats	500 ml
2 cups	low-fat (1% MF) buttermilk	500 ml
1 cup	fresh blueberries	250 ml
2	Granny Smith apples, finely chopped	2
1/4 cup	pecans, chopped	50 ml
2 tbsp	ground flaxseed	25 ml
	maple syrup	
1/4 cup	warm low-fat (1% MF) buttermilk	50 ml
	cinnamon, as garnish	

In a large bowl, combine oats and buttermilk. Cover and refrigerate overnight.

Just before serving, add blueberries, apples, pecans, and flaxseed. Drizzle syrup over oat mixture. Stir in 1/4 cup (50 ml) warm milk per serving. Sprinkle with cinnamon.

Serves 6

Per serving: 267 cal, 10 g pro, 8 g total fat (2 g sat. fat), 41 g carb, 6 g fibre, 5 mg chol, 64 mg sodium

Steamed Quinoa

1 tsp	canola oil	5 ml
1/4 cup	green onions, chopped	50 ml
2 cups	reduced-sodium vegetable stock	500 ml
1 cup	quinoa	250 ml

Heat oil in a saucepan over medium heat, add onions; sauté for 2 to 3 minutes. Add stock and bring to a boil. Stir in quinoa. Reduce heat, cover, and simmer for 12 to 15 minutes or until liquid is absorbed. Remove from heat and fluff with a fork.

Serves 5

Per serving: 170 cal, 6 g pro, 4 g total fat (0 g sat. fat), 29 g carb, 2 g fibre, 1 mg chol, 332 mg sodium

Whole-Wheat Pita Chips

3	6 inch (15 cm) whole-wheat pitas, cut into 6 wedges each	3
	cooking spray	
1/8 tsp	salt	0.5 ml

Preheat oven to 375°F (190°C).

Lightly spray a non-stick baking sheet with cooking spray.

Cut pitas into wedges, place on a baking sheet, and lightly spray with cooking spray. Top with salt. Bake for 8 to 10 minutes or until golden brown and lightly crispy.

Variations: Before baking, sprinkle pita chips with any of the following: ground cumin, paprika, garlic powder, or freshly ground black pepper.

1 serving equals 3 pita chips (equivalent to half of a pita).

Serves 6

Per serving: 98 cal, 3 g pro, 2 g total fat (0 g sat. fat), 18 g carb, 2 g fibre, 0 mg chol, 220 mg sodium

Egg Dishes

Breakfast Burrito

1/2 cup	chopped tomato	125 ml
2 tbsp	finely sliced green onion	25 ml
1	egg	1
	salt and pepper to taste	
1	8 inch (20 cm) whole-wheat fat-free flour tortilla	1
2 tbsp	low-fat salsa	25 ml

Heat skillet over medium heat. Add tomatoes and onion. Cook until vegetables are soft. Add egg, salt, and pepper to skillet and scramble with the vegetables. Cook through, about 4 minutes.

Spread egg mixture over a whole-wheat tortilla. Top with salsa. Fold and serve immediately.

Serves 1

Per serving: 182 cal, 10 g pro, 6 g total fat (2 g sat. fat), 24 g carb, 4 g fibre, 186 mg chol, 266 mg sodium

Breakfast Omelet

	cooking spray	
1/4 cup	diced green bell pepper	50 ml
1 tbsp	chopped chives	15 ml
2	eggs or 4 egg whites	2
	salt and pepper to taste	
1 oz	low-fat cheese, shredded	30 g
	low-fat salsa, as garnish	

Heat a skillet over medium-high heat; coat with cooking spray. Add bell peppers and chives; sauté for 1 minute. Meanwhile, in a small bowl, whisk eggs with salt and pepper until frothy; add to skillet.

Once omelet begins to set, carefully lift the edges with a spatula to allow uncooked portion to flow underneath to the skillet. Cook 3 minutes. Carefully flip omelet, and top with cheese. Cook another 1 to 2 minutes or until set. Slide onto plate and serve with salsa.

Serves 1

Per serving: 220 cal, 20 g pro, 12 g total fat (4 g sat. fat), 7 g carb, 1 g fibre, 378 mg chol, 437 mg sodium

French Toast

1	egg	1
1 tbsp	low-fat milk	15 ml
1 tsp	cinnamon	5 ml
1/4 tsp	pure vanilla extract	1 ml
2	slices whole-grain bread	2

In a shallow dish, whisk egg, milk, cinnamon, and vanilla extract. Dip 2 slices of bread into egg mixture; cook in a non-stick skillet on medium to high heat until lightly browned.

Serves 1

Per serving: 227 cal, 12 g pro, 8 g total fat (2 g sat. fat), 29 g carb, 5 g fibre, 187 mg chol, 368 mg sodium

Smoothies and Fruit

Cranberry Swirl Smoothie

3/4 cup	low-fat yogurt	175 ml
1/2 cup	blueberries	125 ml
1/2 cup	pure cranberry juice	125 ml

In blender, combine yogurt, blueberries, and cranberry juice; purée until thick and frothy.

Serves 1

Per serving: 208 cal, 10 g pro, 1 g total fat (0 g sat. fat), 42 g carbohydrate, 2 g fibre, 3 mg chol, 141 mg sodium

Fresh Fruit Salad

4 cups	assorted fruit (e.g., kiwi, papaya, mango, orange sections, sections, apples, blueberries, strawberries, pineapple)	1 L
1 cup	orange juice	250 ml
2 tsp	lime juice	10 ml
1 tsp	minced gingerroot	5 ml
1 tbsp	chopped fresh mint (optional)	15 ml

In a large bowl, combine fruit, orange juice, lime juice, and ginger. Garnish with chopped mint. Serve cold.

Serves 4

Per serving: 143 cal, 2 g pro, 1 g total fat (0 g sat. fat), 36 g carb, 4 g fibre, 0 mg chol, 5 mg sodium

Friendly Flax Smoothie

1 cup	low-fat milk or calcium-fortified soy milk	250 ml
1/2 cup	mixed berries	125 ml
1/2	banana	1/2
1 tbsp	ground flaxseed	15 ml

In blender, combine milk, berries, banana, and flaxseed; purée until thick and frothy.

Serves 1

Per serving: 225 cal, 10 g pro, 6 g total fat (2 g sat. fat), 35 g carbohydrate, 5 g fibre, 10 mg chol, 127 mg sodium

Mango Tango Smoothie

1 cup	low-fat milk or calcium-fortified soy milk	250 ml
1/2	small mango, sliced	1/2
1/2 cup	pure mango juice	125 ml

In blender, combine milk, mango slices, and mango juice; purée until frothy.

Serves 1

Per serving: 226 cal, 9 g pro, 3 g total fat (2 g sat. fat), 43 g carbohydrate, 3 g fibre, 10 mg chol, 125 mg sodium

Peachy Delight Smoothie

1 cup	low-fat milk or calcium-fortified soy milk	250 ml
1/2 cup	peach slices	125 ml
1/2 cup	pure peach juice	125 ml
1/2 tsp	pure vanilla extract	2 ml

In blender, combine milk, peach slices, peach juice, and vanilla extract; purée until thick and frothy.

Serves 1

Per serving: 212 cal, 10 g pro, 3 g total fat (2 g sat. fat), 38 g carb, 3 g fibre, 10 mg chol, 123 mg sodium

Strawberry Sunrise Smoothie

1 cup	low-fat milk or calcium-fortified soy milk	250 ml
3/4 cup	strawberries	175 ml
1/2	banana	1/2

In blender, combine milk, strawberries, and banana; purée until thick and frothy.

Serves 1

Per serving: 193 cal, 9 g pro, 3 g total fat (2 g sat. fat), 34 g carbohydrate, 4 g fibre, 10 mg chol, 124 mg sodium

Very Berry Smoothie

1/2 cup	low-fat milk or calcium-fortified soy milk	125 ml
1/2 cup	low-fat plain yogurt	125 ml
3/4 cup	strawberries	175 ml
1/2 cup	blueberries	125 ml

In blender, combine milk, yogurt, strawberries, and blueberries; purée until thick and frothy.

Serves 1

Per serving: 192 cal, 11 g pro, 2 g total fat (1 g sat. fat), 34 g carb, 5 g fibre, 7 mg chol, 154 mg sodium

Soups and Salads

Hearty Black Bean Soup

1 tbsp	canola oil	15 ml
1	small onion, chopped	1
3	cloves garlic, minced	3
1/2 cup	chopped celery	125 ml
4 cups	reduced-sodium vegetable or chicken stock	1 L
2	cans (19 oz/540 ml each) black beans, drained and rinsed	2
1/4 cup	chopped cilantro	50 ml
2 tsp	ground cumin	10 ml
	salt and pepper to taste	

In stockpot, heat oil over medium heat. Add onion, garlic, and celery; sauté for 5 minutes or until slightly brown, stirring occasionally. Mix in stock, black beans, cilantro, cumin, salt, and pepper. Bring to a boil, cover and simmer for 20 minutes. Purée soup with a hand blender to desired consistency.

Serves 5

Per serving: 266 cal, 16 g pro, 4 g total fat (1 g sat. fat), 43 g carb, 12 g fibre, 0 mg chol, 645 mg sodium

Hearty Chicken Noodle Soup

1 tsp	canola oil	5 ml
12 oz	skinned, boneless chicken breast halves, cut into 1 inch (2.5 cm) pieces	340 g
1	small onion, chopped	1
2	cloves garlic, minced	2
1 cup	chopped carrot	250 ml
1 cup	chopped celery	250 ml
4 cups	reduced-sodium chicken stock	1 L
1/8 tsp	black pepper, or to taste	0.5 ml
2 cups	chopped spinach	500 ml
2 cups	cooked egg noodles (approx 1 1/2 cups/375 ml uncooked)	500 ml

In a large Dutch oven, heat oil over medium heat. Add chicken; sauté until cooked through. Add onion, garlic, carrot, and celery; sauté for 3 to 4 minutes.

Add stock and pepper; bring to a boil. Cover and simmer for 20 minutes or until cooked through. Just before serving, stir in spinach and egg noodles.

Serves 4

Per serving: 278 cal, 27 g pro, 5 g total fat (1 g sat. fat), 32 g carb, 5 g fibre, 76 mg chol, 1612 mg sodium

Lentil Soup with Turkey Sausage

Add 12 oz (340 g) sliced turkey sausage to Red Pepper Lentil Soup (p. 292), cover, and boil until cooked through.

Serves 6

Per serving: 318 cal, 22 g pro, 8 g total fat (1 g sat. fat), 43 g carb, 6 g fibre, 2 mg chol, 638 mg sodium

Red Pepper Lentil Soup

1 tsp	canola oil	5 ml
2	cloves garlic, minced	2
1/2 cup	chopped carrots	125 ml
1/2 cup	chopped celery	125 ml
1	red bell pepper, chopped	1
1	can (28 oz/796 ml) diced tomatoes	1
1 cup	dried red lentils	250 ml
4 cups	reduced-sodium vegetable stock	1 L
1/2 tsp	each dried basil, oregano, and marjoram	2 ml
1/4 tsp	red pepper flakes	1 ml

In a large saucepan, heat oil over medium heat. Add garlic; sauté until golden brown. Add carrots, celery, bell peppers, tomatoes, lentils, stock, basil, oregano, marjoram, and red pepper flakes; cover and simmer for 20 minutes.

Makes 8 cups

Serves 6

Per serving: 232 cal, 12 g pro, 3 g total fat (1 g sat. fat), 42 g carb, 6 g fibre, 2 mg chol, 604 mg sodium

Salmon Pasta Salad

4 cups	cooked whole-wheat pasta (e.g., rotini, farfalle)	1 L
1/4 cup	lemon juice	50 ml
2 tbsp	chopped fresh dill	25 ml
1 tbsp	olive oil	15 ml
	freshly ground black pepper to taste	
2	cans (7.5 oz/213 g each) salmon, drained	2
1/4 cup	diced red onion	50 ml

Cook pasta according to package directions. Drain and cool.

Whisk together lemon juice, dill, olive oil, and pepper. Combine with cooked pasta, salmon, and red onion in a large bowl. Serve cold.

Serves 4

Per serving: 386 cal, 26 g pro, 15 g total fat (3 g sat. fat), 40 g carb, 4 g fibre, 27 mg chol, 70 mg sodium

Fish

Cajun Fish

1 tsp	each dried thyme, paprika, and garlic powder	5 ml
1/4 tsp	each cayenne and black pepper	1 ml
4	snapper fillets (3 oz/90 g each)	4

Preheat oven to 350°F (180°C).

Mix together thyme, paprika, garlic powder, cayenne pepper, and black pepper. Coat snapper in spice mixture. Place on a non-stick baking sheet and bake for 12 minutes or until fish flakes easily when tested with a fork.

Serves 4

Per serving: 91 cal, 18 g pro, 1 g total fat (0 g sat. fat), 1 g carb, 0 g fibre, 32 mg chol, 55 mg sodium

Citrus Mustard Trout

1/4 cup	lemon juice	50 ml
1 tbsp	honey	15 ml
1 tsp	grainy Dijon mustard	5 ml
1 tsp	canola oil	5 ml
	freshly ground black pepper to taste	
4	rainbow trout fillets (4 oz/120 g each)	4

In a non-stick skillet, combine lemon juice, honey, mustard, oil, and pepper. Add trout; marinate for 20 minutes.

Place skillet over medium heat and cook 5 to 6 minutes per side, or until fish is cooked through and flakes easily when tested with a fork.

Serves 4

Per serving: 134 cal, 18 g pro, 4 g total fat (1 g sat. fat), 7 g carb, 0 g fibre, 49 mg chol, 40 mg sodium

Citrus Soy Salmon

1/4 cup	orange juice	50 ml
1 tbsp	reduced-sodium soy sauce	15 ml
1 tsp	honey	5 ml
1	clove garlic, minced	1
1 tsp	grated gingerroot	5 ml
1 tsp	canola oil	5 ml
4	salmon fillets (3 oz/90 g each)	4

In a non-stick skillet, combine orange juice, soy sauce, honey, garlic, ginger, and oil. Add salmon; marinate for 20 minutes.

Place skillet over medium heat and cook for 5 to 6 minutes per side, or until fish flakes easily when tested with a fork.

Serves 4

Per serving: 182 cal, 17 g pro, 10 g total fat (2 g sat. fat), 4 g carb, 0 g fibre, 50 mg chol, 172 mg sodium

Honey Ginger Tilapia

1/4 cup	lime juice	50 ml
1 tbsp	minced gingerroot	15 ml
1 tbsp	honey	15 ml
1 tsp	grainy Dijon mustard	5 ml
1 tsp	canola oil	5 ml
4	tilapia fillets (3 oz/90 g each)	4

In a non-stick skillet, combine lime juice, ginger, honey, mustard, and oil. Add tilapia; marinate for 20 minutes.

Place skillet over medium heat and cook for 4 to 5 minutes per side, or until fish is cooked through and flakes easily when tested with a fork.

Serves 4

Per serving: 120 cal, 1 g pro, 1 g total fat (1 g sat. fat), 7 g carb, 0 g fibre, 45 mg chol, 15 mg sodium

Lime Cilantro Halibut

3 tbsp	chopped cilantro	50 ml
1/4 cup	lime juice	50 ml
2 tsp	sesame oil	10 ml
1	clove garlic, minced	1
	freshly ground black pepper to taste	
4	halibut fillets (3 oz/90 g each)	4

In a shallow dish, combine cilantro, lime juice, sesame oil, garlic, and pepper. Add halibut; marinate for 20 minutes.

Preheat oven to 375°F (190°C). Place halibut on a non-stick baking sheet and bake for 12 to 16 minutes, or until fish flakes easily when tested with a fork.

Serves 4

Per serving: 118 cal, 18 g pro, 4 g total fat (1 g sat. fat), 1 g carb, 0 g fibre, 27 mg chol, 48 mg sodium

Mango Chutney Salmon—*Quick Start*

4	salmon fillets (4 oz/120 g each)	4
1/3 cup	sweet or hot mango chutney (e.g., Patak's brand)	75 ml
3 tbsp	chopped cilantro	50 ml
1 tsp	canola oil	5 ml

Place salmon in a shallow baking dish and cover with chutney, cilantro, and oil. Let marinate for 20 minutes.

Preheat oven to 350°F (180°C).

Cover baking dish and bake for 12 to 15 minutes, or until fish flakes easily when tested with a fork.

Serves 4

Per serving: 271 cal, 23 g pro, 14 g total fat (3 g sat. fat), 12 g carb, 0 g fibre, 67 mg chol, 68 mg sodium

Maple Glazed Salmon

2 tbsp	reduced-sodium soy sauce	25 ml
1 tbsp	maple syrup	15 ml
2 tsp	grainy Dijon mustard	10 ml
1 tsp	grated gingerroot	5 ml
4	salmon fillets (3 oz/90 g each)	4

In a small bowl, combine soy sauce, maple syrup, mustard, and ginger to make a marinade.

Place the fish in a shallow baking dish, skin side down. Pour marinade over salmon and let stand for 20 minutes.

Preheat oven to 375°F (190°C).

Cover baking dish and bake for 12 to 15 minutes, or until fish flakes easily when tested with a fork.

Serves 4

Per serving: 175 cal, 18 g pro, 9 g total fat (2 g sat. fat), 4 g carb, 0 g fibre, 50 mg chol, 326 mg sodium

Salmon Burgers

1	egg	1
1/2 cup	whole-wheat bread crumbs	125 ml
1 tbsp	ground flaxseed	15 ml
2	cans (7.5 oz/213 g each) salmon, drained	2
1/4 cup	finely chopped onions	50 ml
2 tbsp	chopped fresh dill	25 ml
2 tbsp	lemon juice	25 ml
1 tsp	vegetable oil	5 ml
	salt and pepper to taste	
2	6 inch (15 cm) whole-wheat pita pockets, toasted and cut in half	2
	horseradish, lettuce leaves, sliced tomato, and shredded carrot as garnish	

In a medium-sized bowl, combine egg with bread crumbs and flaxseed until well mixed. Add salmon, onions, dill, lemon juice, oil, salt, and pepper; form into 4 patties.

In a non-stick skillet, heat oil over medium heat. Add salmon patties and cook until golden brown, about 3 to 4 minutes per side. Serve each patty in half a pita pocket, with horseradish, lettuce, sliced tomato, and shredded carrots.

Serves 4

Per serving: 271 cal, 22 g pro, 15 g total fat (3 g sat. fat), 12 g carb, 1 g fibre, 73 mg chol, 198 mg sodium

Sesame Ginger Salmon

1/4 cup	lemon juice	50 ml
1 tbsp	reduced-sodium soy sauce	15 ml
2 tsp	sesame oil	10 ml
1 tsp	lemon zest	5 ml
1 tsp	grated gingerroot	5 ml
1 tsp	honey	5 ml
1	clove garlic, minced	1
4	salmon fillets (3 oz/90g each)	4

In a non-stick skillet, combine lemon juice, soy sauce, oil, lemon zest, ginger, honey, and garlic. Add salmon; marinate for 20 minutes.

Place skillet over medium heat and cook for 4 to 5 minutes per side, or until fish flakes easily when tested with a fork.

Serves 4

Per serving: 189 cal, 17 g pro, 12 g total fat (2 g sat. fat), 4 g carb, 0 g fibre, 50 mg chol, 172 mg sodium

Sesame Soy Trout

2 tbsp	reduced-sodium soy sauce	25 ml
1 tbsp	rice vinegar	15 ml
1 tsp	grated gingerroot	5 ml
1 tsp	sesame oil	5 ml
4	trout fillets (3 oz/90 g each)	4

In a non-stick skillet, combine soy sauce, vinegar, ginger, and oil. Add trout; marinate for 20 minutes.

Place skillet over medium heat and cook for 5 to 6 minutes per side, or until fish flakes easily when tested with a fork.

Serves 4

Per serving: 115 cal, 18 g pro, 4 g total fat (1 g sat. fat), 1 g carb, 0 g fibre, 49 mg chol, 265 mg sodium

Shrimp Stir-Fry

1 tsp	canola oil	5 ml
1	clove garlic, minced	1
2 tsp	grated gingerroot	10 ml
1 cup	red bell pepper, cut into strips	250 ml
1 cup	chopped carrots	250 ml
12 oz	shrimp, peeled and deveined	340 g
2 cups	snow peas	500 ml
2 tbsp	reduced-sodium soy sauce	25 ml
2 tbsp	crushed peanuts	25 ml

In a large non-stick skillet, heat oil over medium heat. Add garlic, ginger, bell peppers, and carrots; stir-fry for 2 minutes. Add shrimp and snow peas; continue to stir-fry for an additional 2 to 3 minutes. Stir in soy sauce and cook 1 minute. Sprinkle with crushed peanuts.

Serves 4

Per serving: 210 cal, 22 g pro, 5 g total fat (1 g sat. fat), 19 g carb, 4 g fibre, 129 mg chol, 392 mg sodium

Sole with Gremolata Sauce

4	sole fillets (3 oz/90 g each)	4
1/2 cup	white wine	125 ml
1/4 cup	chopped fresh parsley	50 ml
1	clove garlic, minced	1
	zest of 1 lemon	
	freshly ground black pepper to taste	

Preheat oven to 375°F (190°C).

In a shallow baking dish, combine sole with wine, parsley, garlic, lemon zest, and pepper. Cover and bake for 15 to 17 minutes, or until fish flakes easily when tested with a fork.

Serves 4

Per serving: 100 cal, 16 g pro, 1 g total fat (0 g sat. fat), 1 g carb, 0 g fibre, 41 mg chol, 73 mg sodium

Tomato Herb Fish—*Quick Start*

4	halibut fillets (4 oz/120 g each)	4
2	tomatoes, diced	2
2	cloves garlic, minced	2
2 tsp	olive oil	10 ml
1/4 tsp	each dried basil, oregano, and thyme	1 ml
1/8 tsp	each salt and pepper	0.5 ml

Preheat oven to 375°F (190°C).

Arrange halibut in a shallow baking dish. Cover with tomatoes, garlic, oil, basil, oregano, thyme, salt, and pepper. Cover and bake for 12 to 15 minutes, or until fish flakes easily when tested with a fork.

Serves 4

Per serving: 161 cal, 24 g pro, 5 g total fat (1 g sat. fat), 4 g carb, 1 g fibre, 36 mg chol, 142 mg sodium

Meat and Poultry

Balsamic Maple Pork Tenderloin

1/4 cup	balsamic vinegar	50 ml
2 tbsp	maple syrup	25 ml
1 tbsp	canola oil	15 ml
1	clove garlic, minced	1
	salt and pepper to taste	
12 oz	pork tenderloin	340 g

In a shallow dish, combine vinegar, maple syrup, oil, garlic, salt, and pepper. Add pork; marinate for 20 to 30 minutes.

Meanwhile, preheat grill to medium. Transfer pork to the grill; cook for 18 to 20 minutes, or until cooked through. Remove pork from grill, cover, and set aside to rest for 5 minutes before serving.

Serves 4

Per serving: 165 cal, 20 g pro, 6 g total fat (1 g sat. fat), 8 g carb, 0 g fibre, 50 mg chol, 44 mg sodium

Beef Curry

1 tsp	canola oil	5 ml
12 oz	lean ground beef	340 g
2	cloves garlic, minced	2
1 tsp	minced gingerroot	5 ml
1	can (28 oz/796 ml) diced tomatoes	1
2 cups	chopped cauliflower florets	500 ml
1 cup	frozen peas	250 ml
1/2 cup	chopped cilantro	125 ml
1 tbsp	curry powder, or to taste	15 ml
1/2 cup	plain low-fat yogurt	125 ml

In a large non-stick skillet, heat oil over medium heat. Add beef; sauté until cooked through. Add garlic and ginger; sauté for 1 minute. Add tomatoes, cauliflower, peas, cilantro, and curry powder. Cover and simmer for 20 minutes.

Remove from heat and cool slightly. Stir in yogurt.

Serves 4

Per serving: 271 cal, 25 g pro, 8 g total fat (3 g sat. fat), 26 g carb, 4 g fibre, 47 mg chol, 571 mg sodium

Chicken Fajitas

Marinade:

2 tbsp	lemon juice	25 ml
2 tbsp	pineapple juice	25 ml
1 tbsp	canola oil	15 ml
1 tsp	red wine vinegar	5 ml
1	clove garlic, minced	1
1 tsp	chili powder	5 ml
1/2 tsp	dried thyme	2 ml

12 oz	boneless chicken breast, cut into strips	340 g
1 tsp	canola oil	5 ml

2	red bell peppers, cut into strips	2
1/2	medium onion, chopped	1/2
8	6 inch (15 cm) soft whole-wheat tortillas	8
	low-fat salsa, fat-free sour cream, lettuce leaves, and chopped tomato, as garnish	

In a shallow bowl, combine lemon juice, pineapple juice, oil, vinegar, garlic, chili powder, and thyme. Add chicken strips; marinate for 30 minutes, or cover and refrigerate overnight.

In non-stick skillet, heat 1 tsp (5 ml) oil over medium heat. Add chicken, bell peppers, and onion, stirring until cooked through.

Serve chicken fajita mixture in whole-wheat soft tortillas with salsa, fat-free sour cream, lettuce, and chopped tomato.

Serves 4

Per serving: 365 cal, 26 g pro, 10 g total fat (2 g sat. fat), 42 g carb, 4 g fibre, 49 mg chol, 342 mg sodium

Chicken Mango Stir-Fry

2 tsp	canola oil	10 ml
12 oz	boneless, skinless chicken breasts, cubed	340 g
1	clove garlic, minced	1
1 tbsp	minced gingerroot	15 ml
2 cups	sliced carrots	500 ml
1 cup	julienne-cut red bell peppers	250 ml
1 cup	snow peas, trimmed	250 ml
1/4 cup	lime juice	50 ml
2 tbsp	reduced-sodium soy sauce	25 ml
1	mango, peeled and sliced	1

In a non-stick skillet, heat oil over medium heat. Add chicken; sauté until cooked through. Add garlic and ginger; sauté for 1 minute.

Add carrots, bell peppers, and snow peas; stir-fry for 2 to 3 minutes, until tender-crisp.

Add lime juice and soy sauce, stirring until heated through; add mango. Serve warm.

Serves 4

Per serving: 242 cal, 23 g pro, 4 g total fat (1 g sat. fat), 30 g carb, 6 g fibre, 49 mg chol, 339 mg sodium

Cumin Citrus Pork

1/4 cup	lime juice	50 ml
1 tsp	honey	5 ml
2	cloves garlic, minced	2
1 tsp	grated gingerroot	5 ml
1 tsp	each ground cumin and ground coriander	5 ml
1 tsp	canola oil	5 ml
12 oz	pork tenderloin	340 g

In a shallow dish, combine lime juice, honey, garlic, ginger, cumin, coriander, and oil. Add pork; marinate for 20 minutes.

Meanwhile, preheat grill to medium. Transfer pork to the grill; cook for 18 to 20 minutes, or until cooked through. Remove pork from grill, cover, and set aside to rest for 5 minutes before serving.

Serves 4

Per serving: 132 cal, 21 g pro, 4 g total fat (1 g sat. fat), 4 g carb, 0 g fibre, 50 mg chol, 44 mg sodium

Curried Chicken Salad Sandwich

12 oz	cooked chicken breast, shredded	340 g
1/4 cup	low-fat plain yogurt	50 ml
1/4 cup	fat-free mayonnaise	50 ml
1/2	apple, finely diced	1/2
2 tbsp	sliced almonds	25 ml
2 tbsp	chopped cilantro (optional)	25 ml
2 tsp	curry powder	10 ml
1 tsp	grated gingerroot	5 ml
2	6 inch (15 cm) whole-wheat pita pockets, cut in half	2

In a medium-sized bowl, combine chicken, yogurt, mayonnaise, apple, almonds, cilantro, curry powder, and ginger. Spread one-quarter of the mixture in half a pita pocket.

Serves 4

Per serving: 270 cal, 25 g pro, 8 g total fat (1 g sat. fat), 25 g carb, 3 g fibre, 50 mg chol, 353 mg sodium

Herbed Pork Tenderloin

1/4 cup	orange juice	50 ml
2 tbsp	canola oil	25 ml
2	cloves garlic, minced	2
1 tbsp	chopped fresh rosemary	15 ml
1 tbsp	chopped fresh thyme	15 ml
	freshly ground black pepper to taste	
12 oz	pork tenderloin, trimmed	340 g

In a shallow dish, combine orange juice, oil, garlic, rosemary, thyme, and pepper. Add pork; marinate for 20 minutes.

Meanwhile, preheat grill to medium. Transfer pork to the grill; cook for 18 to 20 minutes, or until cooked through. Remove pork from grill, cover, and set aside to rest for 5 minutes before serving.

Serves 4

Per serving: 177 cal, 21 g pro, 9 g total fat (1 g sat. fat), 2 g carb, 0 g fibre, 50 mg chol, 43 mg sodium

Honey Garlic Chicken

4	boneless, skinless chicken breasts (3 oz/90 g each)	4
3 tbsp	tomato paste	50 ml
3	cloves garlic, minced	3
2 tbsp	honey	25 ml
1 tbsp	reduced-sodium soy sauce	15 ml
1 tbsp	cider vinegar	15 ml
1/2 tsp	red pepper flakes	2 ml

Preheat oven to 375°F (190°C).

In a baking dish, combine chicken, tomato paste, garlic, honey, soy sauce, vinegar, and red pepper flakes. Cover and bake for 30 to 40 minutes, or until cooked through. Stir chicken once during cooking and add a few tablespoons of water if too dry.

Serves 4

Per serving: 151 cal, 21 g pro, 1 g total fat (0 g sat. fat), 15 g carb, 1 g fibre, 49 mg chol, 192 mg sodium

Honey Glazed Pork Tenderloin—*Quick Start*

2 tbsp	hoisin sauce	25 ml
2 tbsp	reduced-sodium soy sauce	25 ml
1 tbsp	minced gingerroot	15 ml
1 tbsp	apple cider vinegar	15 ml
1 tbsp	honey	15 ml
2 tsp	sesame oil	10 ml
1/4 tsp	black pepper	1 ml
1 lb	pork tenderloin, trimmed	450 g

In a shallow dish, combine hoisin sauce, soy sauce, ginger, vinegar, honey, oil, and pepper. Add pork; marinate for 20 to 30 minutes.

Meanwhile, preheat grill to medium. Transfer pork to the grill; cook for 20 to 22 minutes, or until cooked through. Remove pork from grill, cover, and set aside to rest for 5 minutes before serving.

Serves 4

Per serving: 204 cal, 28 g pro, 5 g total fat (1 g sat. fat), 10 g carb, 0 g fibre, 67 mg chol, 427 mg sodium

Honey Mustard Chicken

3 tbsp	cider vinegar	50 ml
2 tbsp	honey	25 ml
1 tbsp	Dijon mustard	15 ml
1 tsp	canola oil	5 ml
1/4 tsp	dried sage	1 ml
4	boneless, skinless chicken breasts (3 oz/90 g each)	4

In a shallow dish, combine vinegar, honey, mustard, oil, and sage. Add chicken; marinate for 20 minutes.

Meanwhile, preheat grill to medium. Transfer chicken to the grill; cook for 7 to 8 minutes per side, or until cooked through.

Serves 4

Per serving: 147 cal, 20 g pro, 2 g total fat (0 g sat. fat), 11 g carb, 0 g fibre, 49 mg chol, 106 mg sodium

Indian Yogurt Chicken

3/4 cup	low-fat plain yogurt	175 ml
2	cloves garlic, minced	2
2 tbsp	curry powder	25 ml
1 tsp	canola oil	5 ml
1/8 tsp	cayenne pepper	0.5 ml
12 oz	skinless, boneless chicken breast	340 g

Preheat oven to 350°F (180°C).

In a shallow dish, combine yogurt, garlic, curry powder, oil, and cayenne. Add chicken; marinate for 20 minutes.

Cover chicken and bake for 20 to 25 minutes, or until cooked through.

Serves 4

Per serving: 140 cal, 23 g pro, 3 g total fat (1 g sat. fat), 6 g carb, 1 g fibre, 50 mg chol, 90 mg sodium

Jerk Chicken

1 tsp	each ground ginger, garlic powder, and thyme	5 ml
1/2 tsp	each cinnamon and salt	2 ml
1/4 tsp	each ground nutmeg and allspice	1 ml
1/8 tsp	cayenne pepper	0.5 ml
1 tsp	canola oil	5 ml
4	boneless, skinless chicken breasts (3 oz/90 g each)	4

Preheat grill to medium.

In a shallow bowl, combine ginger, garlic powder, thyme, cinnamon, salt, nutmeg, allspice, and cayenne. Lightly oil chicken and pat spice mixture onto chicken breasts.

Grill chicken until cooked through, about 7 to 8 minutes per side.

Serves 4

Per serving: 111 cal, 20 g pro, 2 g total fat (0 g sat. fat), 2 g carb, 0 g fibre, 49 mg chol, 345 mg sodium

Lemon Chicken

1/4 cup	lemon juice	50 ml
1	clove garlic, minced	1
1 tbsp	honey	15 ml
1 tsp	Worcestershire sauce	5 ml
1 tsp	canola oil	5 ml
	zest of 1 lemon	
4	boneless, skinless chicken breasts (3 oz/90 g each)	4

In a shallow baking dish, combine lemon juice, garlic, honey, Worcestershire sauce, oil, and lemon zest. Add chicken; marinate for 20 minutes.

Meanwhile, preheat grill to medium. Transfer chicken to the grill; cook for 7 to 8 minutes per side, or until cooked through.

Serves 4

Per serving: 129 cal, 20 g pro, 2 g total fat (0 g sat. fat), 7 g carb, 0 g fibre, 49 mg chol, 71 mg sodium

Orange Rosemary Chicken

1/4 cup	prepared orange juice	50 ml
1 tbsp	chopped fresh rosemary	15 ml
1	clove garlic, minced	1
1 tsp	canola oil	5 ml
4	3 oz/90 g boneless, skinless chicken breasts	4

In a shallow baking dish, combine orange juice, rosemary, garlic, and oil. Add chicken; marinate for 20 minutes.

Meanwhile, preheat grill to medium. Transfer chicken to the grill; cook for 7 to 8 minutes per side, or until cooked through.

Serves 4

Per serving: 112 cal, 20 g pro, 2 g total fat (0 g sat. fat), 2 g carb, 0 g fibre, 49 mg chol, 56 mg sodium

Rosemary Mustard Chicken—*Quick Start*

1/2 cup	grainy Dijon mustard	125 ml
1/3 cup	lemon juice	75 ml
2 tsp	honey	10 ml
1 tsp	dried rosemary	5 ml
1/4 tsp	black pepper	1 ml
	zest of 1 lemon	
4	boneless, skinless chicken breasts (4 oz/120 g each)	4

In a shallow baking dish, combine mustard, lemon juice, honey, rosemary, pepper, and lemon zest. Add chicken; marinate for 20 minutes.

Meanwhile, preheat grill to medium. Transfer chicken to the grill; cook for 7 to 8 minutes per side, or until cooked through.

Serves 4

Per serving: 172 cal, 27 g pro, 5 g total fat (1 g sat. fat), 4 g carb, 0 g fibre, 66 mg chol, 175 mg sodium

Spaghetti Squash Pasta—*Quick Start*

6 cups	spaghetti squash	1.5 L
2 tbsp	canola oil	25 ml
1 lb	lean ground turkey	450 g
4	cloves garlic, minced	4
1	can (28 oz/796 ml) crushed tomatoes	1
1/4 cup	chopped fresh basil	50 ml
1/4 cup	red wine	50 ml
1/2 tsp	salt	2 ml
1/4 tsp	black pepper	1 ml

Preheat oven to 375°F (190°C).

Cut spaghetti squash in half lengthwise or into quarters. Don't cut it up too small unless you want short strands. Scrape out the seeds and pulp as you would with any winter squash.

Bake rind side up for 30 to 40 minutes. (Or microwave 6 to 8 minutes and let stand for a few minutes afterward.) Separate strands by running a fork through in the "from stem to stern" direction.

Meanwhile, in a large non-stick skillet, heat oil over medium heat. Add ground turkey and cook until it is no longer pink, stirring occasionally. Add garlic; sauté for 1 minute. Add tomatoes, basil, wine, salt, and pepper; bring mixture to a boil. Reduce heat and simmer for 15 minutes.

Serve over cooked spaghetti squash.

Serves 4

Per serving: 354 cal, 26 g pro, 13 g total fat (3 g sat. fat), 36 g carb, 8 g fibre, 90 mg chol, 703 mg sodium

Teriyaki Beef Kabobs

12	bamboo skewers	12
3 tbsp	brown sugar	50 ml
3 tbsp	sherry	50 ml
2 tsp	water	10 ml
2 tsp	reduced-sodium soy sauce	10 ml
2 tsp	canola oil	10 ml
1	clove garlic, minced	1
2 tsp	grated gingerroot	10 ml
12 oz	top sirloin beef, cut into 1 inch (2.5 cm) cubes	340 g
2 cups	red bell peppers, cut into 1 inch (2.5 cm) cubes	500 ml
1 cup	zucchini, cut into 1 inch (2.5 cm) cubes	250 ml
1 cup	mushrooms	250 ml

Soak bamboo skewers in water.

Combine brown sugar, sherry, water, soy sauce, oil, garlic, and ginger to make a marinade. Thread the beef alternately with the bell peppers, zucchini, and mushrooms onto the skewers. Arrange in a shallow baking dish, cover with marinade, and refrigerate for 1 hour, turning occasionally.

Preheat grill to medium. Arrange skewers on grill and cook, turning often, for 12 minutes per side, or until cooked through.

Serves 4

Per serving: 310 cal, 29 g pro, 10 g total fat (3 g sat. fat), 25 g carb, 4 g fibre, 56 mg chol, 142 mg sodium

Teriyaki Sirloin Steak

3 tbsp	brown sugar	50 ml
3 tbsp	sherry	50 ml
2 tsp	water	10 ml
2 tsp	reduced-sodium soy sauce	10 ml
2 tsp	canola oil	10 ml
1	clove garlic, minced	1
2 tsp	grated gingerroot	10 ml
4	sirloin steaks (3 oz/90 g each)	4

In a shallow baking dish, combine brown sugar, sherry, water, soy sauce, oil, garlic, and ginger to make a marinade. Add steaks; marinate for 20 minutes.

Meanwhile, preheat grill to medium. Transfer the steaks to the grill; cook for 6 to 7 minutes per side, or to desired doneness. Use a digital meat thermometer to check temperature of steaks to ensure correct doneness: medium-rare is 145°F (63°C), medium is 160°F (71°C) and well done is 170°F (77°C).

Serves 4

Per serving: 222 cal, 26 g pro, 7 g total fat (2 g sat. fat), 11 g carb, 0 g fibre, 62 mg chol, 141 mg sodium

Thai Peanut Chicken

2 tbsp	light peanut butter	25 ml
1 tbsp	reduced-sodium soy sauce	15 ml
1 tbsp	lime juice	15 ml
2 tsp	sesame oil	10 ml
1	clove garlic, minced	1
1/8 tsp	cayenne pepper	0.5 ml
4	boneless, skinless chicken breasts (3 oz/90 g each)	4

Preheat oven to 375°F (190°C).

In a shallow dish, combine peanut butter, soy sauce, lime juice, oil, garlic, and cayenne. Add chicken; marinate for 20 minutes.

Cover chicken and bake for 20 minutes, or until cooked through.

Serves 4

Per serving: 165 cal, 22 g pro, 7 g total fat (1 g sat. fat), 3 g carb, 1 g fibre, 49 mg chol, 216 mg sodium

Tomato Herb Pasta with Turkey

2 tsp	canola oil	10 ml
12 oz	lean ground turkey	340 g
4	cloves garlic, minced	4
1/4 cup	chopped onions	50 ml
1	can (28 oz/796 ml) crushed tomatoes	1
1/4 cup	chopped fresh basil	50 ml
1/4 cup	red wine	50 ml
1/8 tsp	salt	0.5 ml
1/8 tsp	black pepper	0.5 ml
4 cups	whole-wheat pasta, cooked	1 L

In a large non-stick skillet, heat oil over medium heat. Add ground turkey and cook until it is no longer pink, stirring occasionally. Add garlic and onions; sauté for 1 to 2 minutes. Add tomatoes, basil, wine, salt, and pepper. Reduce heat and simmer for 15 minutes. Serve over cooked whole-wheat pasta.

Serves 4

Per serving: 423 cal, 27 g pro, 11 g total fat (2 g sat. fat), 58 g carb, 10 g fibre, 67 mg chol, 638 mg sodium

Turkey Burgers

12 oz	lean ground turkey	340 g
1/2 cup	whole-wheat bread crumbs	125 ml
1	egg	1
2 tbsp	ground flaxseed	25 ml
2 tbsp	lemon juice	25 ml
1	clove garlic, minced	1
1	green onion, finely chopped	1
1 tsp	chili powder	5 ml
1/4 tsp	dried sage	1 ml
	salt and pepper to taste	

In a medium-sized bowl, combine ground turkey, bread crumbs, egg, flaxseed, lemon juice, garlic, onion, chili powder, sage, salt, and pepper; mix thoroughly. Form mixture into 4 patties. Cook over medium heat in a non-stick skillet for 5 to 6 minutes per side, or until cooked through.

Serves 4

Per serving: 222 cal, 19 g pro, 11 g total fat (3 g sat. fat), 12 g carb, 2 g fibre, 114 mg chol, 219 mg sodium

Turkey Burritos

1 tsp	canola oil	5 ml
2	cloves garlic, minced	2
1	small onion, chopped	1
1	green bell pepper, cut into strips	1
1 lb	lean ground turkey	450 g
1	can (19 oz/540 ml) black beans, drained and rinsed	1
1	pkg prepared burrito seasoning	1
	water	
6	10 inch (25 cm) whole-wheat soft tortilla shells	6
	low-fat salsa, chopped tomato, and shredded lettuce, as garnish	

In a non-stick skillet, heat oil over medium heat. Add garlic, onion, and bell peppers; sauté until lightly brown. Add ground turkey; sauté, stirring often until turkey is cooked through.

Add black beans, seasoning, and water according to seasoning package directions. Cover and simmer until slightly thickened.

Serve in whole-wheat tortilla shells with low-fat salsa, chopped tomato, and shredded lettuce.

Serves 6

Per serving: 511 cal, 27 g pro, 13 g total fat (3 g sat. fat), 69 g carb, 9 g fibre, 60 mg chol, 659 mg sodium

Turkey Chili

1 tbsp	vegetable oil	15 ml
1/2 cup	chopped celery	125 ml
1/4 cup	chopped onions	50 ml
2	cloves garlic, minced	2
1 lb	lean ground turkey	450 g
1	can (28 oz/796 ml) diced tomatoes	1
1	can (19 oz/540 ml) kidney beans, drained and rinsed	1
1	can (19 oz/540 ml) black beans, drained and rinsed	1
3 tbsp	chili powder, or to taste	50 ml
1 tsp	ground cumin	5 ml
1/4 tsp	cayenne pepper, or to taste	1 ml

In a non-stick pan, heat oil over medium heat. Add celery, onions, and garlic. Cook for 3 to 4 minutes, or until golden, stirring occasionally. Add turkey; sauté until cooked through.

Add tomatoes, kidney and black beans, chili powder, cumin, and cayenne. Cover and simmer for 30 minutes. Serve warm.

Serves 6

Per serving: 371 cal, 27 g pro, 10 g total fat (2 g sat. fat), 45 g carb, 12 g fibre, 60 mg chol, 437 mg sodium

Turkey Lasagna

1 lb	lean ground turkey	450 g
2	cloves garlic, minced	2
1	onion, chopped	1
1	jar (24 oz/700 ml) low-fat commercial pasta sauce	1
2 tsp	dried oregano	10 ml
1 tsp	dried basil	5 ml
1/4 tsp	black pepper	1 ml
	cooking spray	
12	cooked whole-wheat lasagna noodles	12
1	tub (18 oz/500 g) fat-free cottage cheese	1
1	pkg (10 oz/300 g) frozen spinach leaves, thawed	1
1 cup	reduced-fat shredded mozzarella	250 ml

In a non-stick skillet, cook turkey over medium heat until brown, adding water as necessary to prevent sticking. Add garlic and onion; continue to cook for 2 to 3 minutes. Stir in pasta sauce, oregano, basil, and pepper; cover and simmer for 10 minutes.

Preheat oven to 350°F (180°C).

Coat a 13 x 9 inch (3.5 L) baking dish with cooking spray. Spread one-quarter of the meat mixture in bottom of dish. Arrange 4 noodles over meat mixture and top with half of the cottage cheese, half of the spinach, 1/4 cup (50 ml) meat mixture, and 1/3 cup (75 ml) cheese.

Repeat layers, topping with noodles. Spread remaining meat mixture over noodles. Cover and bake at 350°F (180°C) for 45 minutes. Uncover and sprinkle with remaining mozzarella cheese; bake until cheese begins to melt, about 5 minutes.

Note: If lasagna seems dry when cooking, pour 1 cup (250 ml) water over lasagna.

Serves 9

Per serving: 373 cal, 34 g pro, 10 g total fat (4 g sat. fat), 38 g carb, 6 g fibre, 57 mg chol, 802 mg sodium

Legumes and Soy

Chickpea Burgers

2 tsp	olive oil	10 ml
1	small onion, chopped	1
2	cloves garlic, minced	2
1	can (19 oz/540 ml) chickpeas, drained and rinsed	1
1/3 cup	whole-wheat bread crumbs	75 ml
1	egg	1
1 tbsp	ground flaxseed	15 ml
2 tbsp	lemon juice	25 ml
1/2 tsp	salt	2 ml
1/8 tsp	black pepper	0.5 ml
1/8 tsp	cayenne pepper	0.5 ml

In a non-stick skillet, heat 1 tsp (5 ml) oil over medium heat. Add onion and garlic; sauté for 1 to 2 minutes, or until lightly brown. Cool.

In a food processor, pulse chickpeas and onion mixture until coarse. Turn into a medium-sized bowl and add bread crumbs, egg, flaxseed, lemon juice, salt, black pepper, and cayenne. Mix well.

Form mixture into 4 large patties or 8 small patties.

In a non-stick skillet, heat remaining 1 tsp (5 ml) oil over medium heat; add patties and cook until lightly brown, about 4 minutes per side.

Serve on whole-grain rolls.

Serves 4

Per serving: 257 cal, 12 g pro, 7 g total fat (1 g sat. fat), 37 g carb, 6 g fibre, 47 mg chol, 389 mg sodium

Marinated Tofu

1/4 cup	lemon juice	50 ml
2 tbsp	reduced-sodium soy sauce	25 ml
1 tsp	minced gingerroot	5 ml
1 tsp	honey	5 ml
1	clove garlic, minced	1
1 1/2 cups	extra-firm tofu, cut into 1/2 inch (12 mm) slices	375 ml

In a non-stick skillet, combine lemon juice, soy sauce, ginger, honey, and garlic. Add tofu; marinate for 20 minutes. Heat over medium heat, until tofu begins to brown. Remove from heat and serve warm.

Serves 2

Per serving: 305 cal, 31 g pro, 17 g total fat (2 g sat. fat), 16 g carb, 2 g fibre, 0 mg chol, 511 mg sodium

Mexican Bean Salad

1	can (19 oz/540 ml) black beans, drained and rinsed	1
1	can (19 oz/540 ml) kidney beans, drained and rinsed	1
1	can (19 oz/540 ml) chickpeas, drained and rinsed	1
2	large tomatoes, chopped	2
Dressing:		
3/4 cup	loosely packed chopped cilantro	175 ml
1/2 cup	lime juice	125 ml
3	cloves garlic, minced	3
4	green onions, finely chopped	4
1 tbsp	olive oil	15 ml
1/2 tsp	red pepper flakes	2 ml

In a large bowl, mix together black beans, kidney beans, chickpeas, and tomatoes.

In a separate bowl, whisk together cilantro, lime juice, garlic, onions, oil, and red pepper flakes. Toss beans and tomatoes with dressing.

Cover and refrigerate the salad for at least 2 hours before serving.

Serves 8

Per serving: 243 cal, 14 g pro, 4 g total fat (0 g sat. fat), 41 g carb, 10 g fibre, 0 mg chol, 11 mg sodium

Moroccan Chickpea Stew

1 tbsp	canola oil	15 ml
1	small onion, chopped	1
2	cloves garlic, minced	2
2 cups	cubed sweet potatoes	500 ml
1 cup	sliced carrots	250 ml
1/2 cup	chopped celery	125 ml
1	can (19 oz/540 ml) chickpeas, drained and rinsed	1
1	can (28 oz/796 ml) diced tomatoes	1
1/4 cup	dried apricots	50 ml
1/4 cup	raisins	50 ml
1 tsp	cinnamon	5 ml
1/2 tsp	each ground ginger, turmeric, and nutmeg	2 ml
1	bay leaf	1

In a large skillet, heat oil over medium heat. Add onion and garlic; sauté until lightly brown. Add sweet potatoes, carrots, celery, chickpeas, tomatoes, apricots, raisins, cinnamon, ginger, turmeric, nutmeg, and bay leaf. Cover and simmer for 45 minutes. Serve warm.

Makes 8 cups (2 L)

Serves 5

Per serving: 353 cal, 10 g pro, 5 g total fat (1 g sat. fat), 73 g carb, 12 g fibre, 0 mg chol, 754 mg sodium

Sesame Tofu Stir-Fry—*Quick Start*

2 tsp	sesame oil	10 ml
2	cloves garlic, minced	2
1 tbsp	minced gingerroot	15 ml
1	pkg (12 oz/350 g) extra-firm tofu, cubed	1
3 cups	chopped assorted vegetables (e.g., carrots, snow peas, broccoli, peppers)	750 ml
1 cup	bok choy, trimmed	250 ml
1/4 cup	reduced-sodium soy sauce	50 ml
1 tbsp	cornstarch	15 ml
1 tbsp	rice vinegar	15 ml
2 tsp	toasted sesame seeds	10 ml

In a large wok, heat oil over medium heat. Add garlic and ginger; sauté for 1 minute. Add tofu, chopped vegetables, and bok choy; sauté for 4 to 5 minutes, until tender-crisp.

In a small bowl, combine soy sauce, cornstarch, and vinegar. Pour over vegetables and tofu; heat until sauce thickens slightly. Remove from heat; sprinkle with sesame seeds. Serve warm.

Serves 4

Per serving: 260 cal, 20 g pro, 11 g total fat (2 g sat. fat), 27 g carb, 6 g fibre, 0 mg chol, 559 mg sodium

Sweet and Sour Tofu Stir-Fry

1	can (20 oz/590 ml) pineapple tidbits, drained, reserving 2/3 cup (150 ml) of juice	1
1/4 cup	cider vinegar	50 ml
2 tbsp	reduced-sodium soy sauce	25 ml
1 tsp	honey	5 ml
1	pkg (12 oz/350 g) extra-firm tofu, cubed	1
1 tbsp	cornstarch	15 ml
2 tsp	canola oil	10 ml
2	cloves garlic, minced	2
2 tsp	grated gingerroot	10 ml
1 cup	red bell pepper, cut into strips	250 ml
1 cup	snow peas, trimmed	250 ml
1 cup	sliced carrots	250 ml

Alternatively, use 3 cups (1 L) assorted frozen Asian vegetables in place of those listed.

Drain pineapple and set aside, reserving 2/3 cup (150 ml) of the juice. In a small bowl, combine reserved pineapple juice, vinegar, soy sauce, and honey to make a marinade.

Place tofu cubes in a shallow dish, cover with 1/4 cup (50 ml) of the marinade, and let stand for 20 minutes. Add the cornstarch to the remaining marinade and whisk until blended.

In a non-stick skillet, heat 1 tsp (5 ml) oil over medium-high heat. Add tofu, stirring often until lightly brown, about 6 minutes. Remove tofu from pan.

Heat remaining 1 tsp (5 ml) oil in the same skillet. Add garlic and ginger; sauté for 1 minute. Add bell peppers, snow peas, and carrots; cook, stirring often, until tender-crisp, about 3 to 4 minutes.

Pour in marinade and heat until slightly thickened. Add tofu and pineapple and cook until heated through, about 2 to 3 minutes.

Serves 3

Per serving: 435 cal, 23 g pro, 14 g total fat (2 g sat. fat), 64 g carb, 8 g fibre, 0 mg chol, 371 mg sodium

Tofu Vegetable Stir-Fry

1 tbsp	canola oil	15 ml
2	cloves garlic, minced	2
1 tbsp	minced gingerroot	15 ml
1	pkg (12 oz/350 g) extra-firm tofu, cubed	1
1 cup	chopped broccoli	250 ml
1 cup	sliced carrots	250 ml
1 cup	chopped celery	250 ml
1/2 cup	snow peas, trimmed	125 ml
1/2 cup	sliced mushrooms	125 ml
1/2 cup	reduced-sodium vegetable stock	125 ml
2 tbsp	reduced-sodium soy sauce	25 ml
1 tbsp	cornstarch	15 ml
1	green onion, chopped, as garnish	1

In a skillet, heat oil over medium heat. Add garlic and ginger; sauté for 1 minute. Add tofu, broccoli, carrots, celery, snow peas, and mushrooms; continue to cook, stirring, for 3 to 4 minutes.

In a small bowl, combine stock, soy sauce, and cornstarch.

Pour stock mixture over the stir-fry; heat until the sauce in the pan begins to thicken. Remove from heat. Garnish with chopped green onion.

Serves 4

Per serving: 390 cal, 35 g pro, 20 g total fat (3 g sat. fat), 29 g carb, 8 g fibre, 0 mg chol, 457 mg sodium

Tomato Herb Pasta with Veggie Ground Round

2 tsp	canola oil	10 ml
12 oz	veggie ground round (e.g., 1 pkg of Yves)	340 g
4	cloves garlic, minced	4
1/4 cup	chopped onions	50 ml
1	can (28 oz/796 ml) crushed tomatoes	1
1/4 cup	chopped fresh basil	50 ml
1/4 cup	red wine	50 ml
1/8 tsp	salt	0.5 ml
1/8 tsp	black pepper	0.5 ml
4 cups	whole-wheat pasta, cooked	1 L

In a large non-stick skillet, heat oil over medium heat. Add veggie ground round; cook until heated through, stirring occasionally. Add garlic and onions; sauté for 1 to 2 minutes. Add tomatoes, basil, wine, salt, and pepper. Reduce heat and simmer for 15 minutes. Serve over cooked whole-wheat pasta.

Serves 4

Per serving: 389 cal, 27 g pro, 5 g total fat (0 g sat. fat), 66 g carb, 13 g fibre, 0 mg chol, 558 mg sodium

Vegetarian Chili

1 tbsp	vegetable oil	15 ml
1/2 cup	chopped celery	125 ml
1/4 cup	chopped onions	50 ml
2	cloves garlic, minced	2
18 oz	veggie ground round (e.g., 1 1/2 pkg of Yves)	510 g
1	can (28 oz/796 ml) diced tomatoes	1
1	can (19 oz/540 ml) kidney beans, drained and rinsed	1
1	can (19 oz/540 ml) black beans, drained and rinsed	1
3 tbsp	chili powder, or to taste	50 ml
1 tsp	ground cumin	5 ml
1/4 tsp	cayenne pepper, or to taste	1 ml

In a non-stick pan, heat oil over medium heat. Add celery, onions, and garlic. Cook for 3 to 4 minutes, or until golden, stirring occasionally. Add veggie ground round; sauté until heated through.

Add tomatoes, kidney beans, black beans, chili powder, cumin, and cayenne. Cover and simmer for 30 minutes. Serve warm.

Serves 6

Per serving: 351 cal, 30 g pro, 5 g total fat (1 g sat. fat), 53 g carb, 15 g fibre, 0 mg chol, 366 mg sodium

White Bean Dip

1	can (19 oz/540 ml) white beans (white kidney or cannellini), drained and rinsed	1
2	cloves garlic, minced	2
1/4 cup	chopped parsley	50 ml
2 tbsp	olive oil	25 ml
2 tbsp	lemon juice	25 ml
1 tbsp	chopped fresh thyme	15 ml
	salt and pepper to taste	

Combine beans, garlic, parsley, oil, lemon juice, thyme, salt, and pepper in a food processor; pulse until smooth.

Cover and refrigerate until ready to serve.

Serve with Whole-Wheat Pita Chips (p. 285).

Tip: If dip is too thick, add an additional teaspoon (5 ml) lemon juice.

Serves 6

Per serving: 133 cal, 6 g pro, 5 g total fat (0 g sat. fat), 17 g carb, 0 g fibre, 0 mg chol, 3 mg sodium

Whole-Grain Lentil Casserole

1 1/2 cups	reduced-sodium vegetable or chicken stock	375 ml
1/2 cup	dried green or brown lentils	125 ml
1/2 cup	uncooked brown rice	125 ml
1 cup	stewed tomatoes	250 ml
1/2 cup	dry white wine or lemon juice	125 ml
1	medium onion, chopped	1
1	clove garlic, minced	1
1/4 tsp	dried thyme	1 ml
1/4 tsp	dried basil	1 ml
1	bay leaf	1
	salt and pepper to taste	
1/2 cup	reduced-fat shredded cheese, such as mozzarella	125 ml

Preheat oven to 350°F (180°C).

In a 6 cup (1.5 L) casserole dish, combine stock, lentils, rice, tomatoes, wine or lemon juice, onion, garlic, thyme, basil, bay leaf, salt, and pepper.

Cover with foil and bake for 1 1/2 hours, stirring 2 or 3 times. Sprinkle cheese on top and bake for another 5 minutes.

Serves 4

Per serving: 243 cal, 11 g pro, 3 g total fat (0 g sat. fat), 41 g carb, 5 g fibre, 0 mg chol, 730 mg sodium

Vegetables

Balsamic Roasted Asparagus

1	large bunch asparagus, washed and trimmed	1
2 tbsp	balsamic vinegar	25 ml
1 tsp	olive oil	5 ml
	salt and pepper to taste	

Preheat oven to 375°F (190°C).

Lay asparagus on a baking sheet; drizzle with vinegar and oil. Sprinkle with salt and pepper. Bake for 15 to 20 minutes or until tender.

Serves 4

Per serving: 107 cal, 10 g pro, 2 g total fat (0 g sat. fat), 19 g carb, 6 g fibre, 0 mg chol, 8 mg sodium

Lemon Swiss Chard

1 tsp	canola oil	5 ml
1	clove garlic, minced	1
1	large bunch Swiss chard, washed and trimmed (about 6 cups/1.5 L)	1
1 tbsp	lemon juice	15 ml
	salt and pepper to taste	

In a large skillet, heat oil over medium heat. Add garlic; sauté until golden brown. Add Swiss chard; cover and steam for several minutes, until the chard is wilted. Remove from heat, sprinkle with lemon juice, salt, and pepper. Serve warm.

Serves 4

Per serving: 22 cal, 1 g pro, 1 g total fat (0 g sat. fat), 2 g carb, 1 g fibre, 0 mg chol, 116 mg sodium

Pepper and Snow Pea Sauté

1 tsp	canola oil	5 ml
1	clove garlic	1
1 tsp	minced gingerroot	5 ml
2 cups	green, red and yellow bell peppers, cut into strips	500 ml
2 cups	snow peas, trimmed	500 ml
1 tbsp	balsamic vinegar	15 ml

In a non-stick skillet, heat oil over medium heat. Add garlic and ginger; sauté for 1 minute. Add bell peppers and snow peas; sauté for 2 to 3 minutes. Remove from heat, drizzle with balsamic vinegar.

Serves 4

Per serving: 83 cal, 3 g pro, 2 g total fat (0 g sat. fat), 16 g carb, 3 g fibre, 0 mg chol, 6 mg sodium

Sweet Potato Wedges

2	medium sweet potatoes	2
2 tsp	canola oil	10 ml
1 tsp	ground cumin	5 ml
	salt and pepper to taste	

Preheat oven to 375°F (190°C).

Cut sweet potatoes into finger-like wedges. Whisk together oil and cumin; coat potato wedges. Arrange wedges on a non-stick baking sheet; bake for 30 to 40 minutes, or until tender.

Serves 4

Per serving: 199 cal, 2 g pro, 3 g total fat (0 g sat. fat), 42 g carb, 6 g fibre, 0 mg chol, 14 mg sodium

Veggie Stir-Fry

2 tbsp	orange juice concentrate	25 ml
1 tbsp	reduced-sodium soy sauce	15 ml
2 tsp	cornstarch	10 ml
1 tsp	sesame oil	5 ml
1 tsp	canola oil	5 ml
2	cloves garlic, minced	2
1 tsp	minced gingerroot	5 ml
4 cups	chopped assorted vegetables (e.g., broccoli, carrots)	1 L

In a small bowl, whisk together orange juice concentrate, soy sauce, cornstarch, and sesame oil.

In a non-stick skillet, heat canola oil over medium heat. Add garlic, ginger, and vegetables; sauté for 2 to 3 minutes. Add soy sauce mixture, stirring until sauce is heated through and thickened.

Serves 4

Per serving: 151 cal, 6 g pro, 3 g total fat (0 g sat. fat), 29 g carb, 5 g fibre, 0 mg chol, 185 mg sodium

Low-Fat Dressings and Marinades

Honey Lemon Dressing

4 tbsp	lemon juice	50 ml
3 tbsp	olive oil	40 ml
1 tsp	ground flaxseed	5 ml
2 tsp	Worcestershire sauce	10 ml
2 tsp	Dijon mustard	10 ml
2 tsp	honey	10 ml

In a small bowl, combine lemon juice, oil, flaxseed, Worcestershire sauce, mustard, and honey. Keep refrigerated for up to 5 days.

Serves 6

Per serving: 75 cal, 0 g pro, 7 g total fat (1 g sat. fat), 4 g carb, 0 g fibre, 0 mg chol, 43 mg sodium

Italian Vinaigrette

1/4 cup	olive oil	50 ml
1/4 cup	reduced-sodium vegetable stock	50 ml
1/4 cup	balsamic vinegar	50 ml
1 tbsp	Dijon mustard	15 ml
1 tsp	honey	5 ml
1/4 tsp	each dried basil and oregano	1 ml

In a small bowl, combine oil, stock, vinegar, mustard, honey, basil, and oregano; mix well. Keep refrigerated for up to 5 days.

Serves 6

Per serving: 63 cal, 0 g pro, 7 g total fat (1 g sat. fat), 1 g carb, 0 g fibre, 0 mg chol, 46 mg sodium

Orange Ginger Dressing

2 tbsp	orange juice	25 ml
1 tbsp	honey	15 ml
1 tbsp	olive oil	15 ml
2 tsp	white wine vinegar	10 ml
1 tsp	Dijon mustard	5 ml
1 tsp	minced gingerroot	5 ml
1/4 tsp	freshly ground black pepper	1 ml

In a small bowl, combine orange juice, honey, oil, vinegar, mustard, ginger, and pepper; mix well. Keep refrigerated for up to 5 days.

Serves 6

Per serving: 36 cal, 0 g pro, 2 g total fat (0 g sat. fat), 4 g carb, 0 g fibre, 0 mg chol, 11 mg sodium

Poppy Seed Dressing

1/2 cup	plain low-fat yogurt	125 ml
2 tsp	orange juice concentrate	10 ml
2 tsp	honey	10 ml
1 tsp	poppy seeds	5 ml

In a small bowl, combine yogurt, orange juice concentrate, honey, and poppy seeds. Serve over spinach salad.

Serves 4

Per serving: 37 cal, 2 g pro, 0 g total fat (0 g sat. fat), 7 g carb, 0 g fibre, 1 mg chol, 22 mg sodium

Sesame Miso Dressing

2 tbsp	miso (soybean paste)	25 ml
2 tbsp	seasoned rice vinegar	25 ml
1 tbsp	minced gingerroot	15 ml
1 tsp	toasted sesame seeds	5 ml
1 tsp	sesame oil	5 ml
1/2 tsp	Dijon mustard	2 ml
1/2 tsp	honey	2 ml

In a small bowl, combine miso, vinegar, ginger, sesame seeds, sesame oil, mustard, and honey; mix well. Keep refrigerated for up to 5 days.

Serves 6

Per serving: 25 cal, 1 g pro, 1 g total fat (0 g sat. fat), 3 g carb, 1 g fibre, 0 mg chol, 215 mg sodium

Thai Peanut Sauce Marinade

2 tbsp	light peanut butter	25 ml
1 tbsp	reduced-sodium soy sauce	15 ml
1 tbsp	lime juice	15 ml
2 tsp	sesame oil	10 ml
1	clove garlic, minced	1
1/8 tsp	cayenne pepper	0.5 ml

In a small bowl, combine peanut butter, soy sauce, lime juice, sesame oil, garlic, and cayenne pepper; mix well.

This marinade works well with chicken and tofu.

Teriyaki Marinade

3 tbsp	brown sugar	50 ml
3 tbsp	sherry	50 ml
2 tsp	grated gingerroot	10 ml
2 tsp	water	10 ml
2 tsp	reduced-sodium soy sauce	10 ml
2 tsp	canola oil	10 ml
1	clove garlic, minced	1

In a small bowl, combine sugar, sherry, ginger, water, soy sauce, oil, and garlic; mix well.

This marinade works well with fish, pork, and beef.

Sesame Ginger Marinade

1/4 cup	lemon juice	50 ml
1 tbsp	reduced-sodium soy sauce	15 ml
2 tsp	sesame oil	10 ml
1 tsp	lemon zest	5 ml
1 tsp	grated gingerroot	5 ml
1 tsp	honey	5 ml
1	clove garlic, minced	1

In a small bowl, combine lemon juice, soy sauce, sesame oil, lemon zest, ginger, honey, and garlic; mix well.

This marinade works well with fish, chicken, and tofu.

Honey Glaze Marinade

2 tbsp	hoisin sauce	25 ml
2 tbsp	reduced-sodium soy sauce	25 ml
1 tbsp	minced gingerroot	15 ml
1 tbsp	apple cider vinegar	15 ml
1 tbsp	honey	15 ml
2 tsp	sesame oil	10 ml
1/4 tsp	freshly ground black pepper	1 ml

In a small bowl, combine hoisin sauce, soy sauce, ginger, vinegar, honey, sesame oil, and black pepper; mix well.

This marinade works well with fish and pork.

Balsamic Maple Marinade

1/4 cup	balsamic vinegar	50 ml
2 tbsp	maple syrup	25 ml
1 tbsp	canola oil	15 ml
1	clove garlic, minced	1
	salt and pepper to taste	

In a small bowl, combine vinegar, maple syrup, oil, garlic, salt and pepper; mix well.

This marinade works well with pork.

Appendix 1
Tracking Tools

The No-Fail Diet Daily Food and Activity Tracker

Meal/Snack	Foods Eaten	Portion Size	Number of No-Fail Diet Food Group Servings
Breakfast Time: _____			
Snack Time: _____			
Lunch Time: _____			
Snack Time: _____			
Dinner Time: _____			

Activity Tracker

What did you do? (Include all daily physical activity such as walking and stair climbing as well as planned exercise.)

_____

Activity   **Number of minutes' duration**

_____

Activity   **Number of minutes' duration**

_____

Activity   **Number of minutes' duration**

_____

Activity   **Number of minutes' duration**

_____

Activity   **Number of minutes' duration**

_____

Assessing Your Food and Activity

Each day, take a moment to reflect on what you wrote down by answering the following questions:

Did I apply the factors of the No-Fail Diet?

I included protein at each meal.   Yes ☐   No ☐
If no, why not? _____
_____
_____
_____

I ate every 3 to 4 hours.   Yes ☐   No ☐
If no, why not? _____
_____
_____
_____

I monitored my portion sizes.   Yes ☐   No ☐
If no, why not? _____
_____
_____
_____

Did I reach my daily target for Food Group Servings?
(Check one box per serving.)

(Depending on the calorie level of your Phase 2 meal plan, all boxes may not need to be checked.)

Protein Foods ☐ ☐ ☐ ☐ ☐ ☐ ☐ ☐
Milk and Milk Alternatives ☐ ☐ ☐
Starchy Foods ☐ ☐ ☐ ☐ ☐ ☐ ☐
Fruit ☐ ☐ ☐
Vegetables ☐ ☐ ☐ ☐ ☐ ☐ ☐ ☐ ☐ ☐
Fats and Oils ☐ ☐ ☐ ☐ ☐ ☐
Water (cups) ☐ ☐ ☐ ☐ ☐ ☐ ☐ ☐ ☐ ☐ ☐ ☐ ☐
(Targets: 9 cups/2.2 litres for women, 13 cups/3 litres for men)

Did I drink any alcoholic beverages?

Yes ☐   No ☐   How many? _____

(Weekly upper limit: seven drinks for women, nine drinks for men.)

Did I eat anything off my plan?

Yes ☐   No ☐   What? _____

_____

_____

_____

_____

(One treat or splurge per week is allowed on Phase 2.)

Did I rate my hunger level before, halfway through, and after eating my meals?

Yes ☐   No ☐   What did I learn? _____

_____

_____

_____

_____

Did I plan my meals and snacks in advance?

Yes ☐   No ☐

Did a lack of planning influence my food choices or how much I ate?

Yes ☐   No ☐

Did I notice any emotions that prompted me to eat when I was not hungry?

Yes ☐   No ☐   If so, what were they? _____

_____

_____

_____

_____

_____

How can I prevent these emotions from influencing my food intake tomorrow?

_____

_____

_____

_____

_____

_____

_____

_____

_____

_____

_____

_____

_____

_____

_____

What will I do differently tomorrow, if anything?

1._____

_____

_____

2._____

_____

_____

3._____

_____

_____

4._____

_____

_____

_____

The No-Fail Diet 12-Week Body Measurement Tracker

Record your weight once each week, on the same day of the week and in the morning.

Other body measurements are to be taken once per month. To learn how to take your measurements correctly, and how to calculate your body mass index and waist-to-hip ratio, see pages 21 to 23 in Chapter 1.

Your measurements	Week 1	Week 2	Week 3	Week 4	Week 5	Week 6
Weight (lbs or kg)						
Body Mass Index (BMI)						
Chest/Bust (inches)						
Waist (inches)						
Hips (inches)						
Waist-to-Hip Ratio (WHR)						

	Week 7	Week 8	Week 9	Week 10	Week 11	Week 12
Weight (lbs or kg)						
Body Mass Index (BMI)						
Chest/Bust (inches)						
Waist (inches)						
Hips (inches)						
Waist-to-Hip Ratio (WHR)						

The No-Fail Diet 12-Week Fitness Tracker

Weeks 1, 2, and 3

If you are following the No-Fail 12-Week Fitness Program outlined in Chapter 5 (and I encourage you to do so), use this tracking form to monitor your fitness-level progress.

Program components	Week 1	Week 2	Week 3
• Standard Cardio			
Number of workouts			
Duration (minutes)			
• Interval Cardio (duration)			
• Extended Cardio (duration)			
• 7 Stretches completed after cardio			
• Strength training			
Number of workouts			
• Upper body workouts (amount of weight lifted)			
Bicep curl			
Overhead triceps			
Lat pull down			
Chest fly			

Weeks 4, 5, and 6

Program Components	Week 4	Week 5	Week 6
• Standard Cardio			
Number of workouts			
Duration (minutes)			
• Interval Cardio (duration)			
• Extended Cardio (duration)			
• 7 Stretches completed after cardio?			
• Strength training			
Number of workouts			
• Upper body workouts (amount of weight lifted)			
Hammer curl			
Triceps kickback			
Chest press			
Standing forward row			

Weeks 7, 8, and 9

Program Components	Week 7	Week 8	Week 9
• Standard Cardio			
Number of workouts			
Duration (minutes)			
• Interval Cardio (duration)			
• Extended Cardio (duration)			
• 7 Stretches completed after cardio?			
• Strength training			
Number of workouts			
• Upper body workouts (amount of weight lifted)			
Chest fly on exercise ball			
Seated forward row			
Chest squeeze			
Bent over fly			

Weeks 10, 11, and 12

Program Components	Week 10	Week 11	Week 12
• Standard Cardio			
Number of workouts			
Duration (minutes)			
• Interval Cardio (duration)			
• Extended Cardio (duration)			
• 7 Stretches completed after cardio?			
• Strength training			
Number of workouts			
• Upper body workouts (amount of weight lifted)			
Bicep concentration curl			
Triceps dip (number done)			
Lateral lift			
Anterior lift			

Appendix 2
Frequently Asked Questions

Meal Timing

What happens if I miss a meal? May I eat more at the next meal?

Ideally, you don't want to a skip meal because you'll end up being overly hungry at your next meal and more likely to overeat. However, there will be times when, because of unforeseen events, you can't help missing a meal. If this happens, make sure to eat your planned between-meal snack. If you're going to be away from home for a few hours at a time, always take your snack with you.

If you do miss a meal, you may move 2 food group servings (e.g., 1 Protein Food serving and 1 Starchy Food serving) from the meal you missed to your snack. This will help keep you feeling satisfied until your next meal.

Should I eat before or after exercise?

That depends on what time you plan to work out, and what type of workout you plan to do. If you are doing a cardio workout first thing in the morning, you don't need to eat anything before you exercise. You'll eat your breakfast after you've finished. If you plan to work out with weights, however, I do recommend that you eat part of your breakfast (e.g., 1 Fruit Serving or 1 Milk and Milk Alternative serving) before you hit the gym. If you are exercising at noon, have your mid-morning snack at the usual time and then eat lunch after your workout. If you are exercising after work, have your planned after-noon snack, and then eat dinner after your workout.

Eating Away from Home

If I am going to a restaurant for dinner, should I skip breakfast and lunch to compensate for the extra calories I am bound to eat?

Definitely not. Saving all your calories for one big meal will only cause you to feel ravenous by the time you arrive at the restaurant. You'll end up devouring all the bread in the basket before your meal arrives! Always eat your full breakfast. However, you may choose to move some of your Starchy Food servings or Fats and Oils servings from lunch to dinner. But your lunch must include protein. And be sure to eat your planned afternoon snack. This will help keep your appetite in check at the restaurant.

How do I order healthfully in restaurants?

I don't expect you to eat all your meals at home while losing weight on the No-Fail Diet. If you will be dining out, plan in advance which restaurant you will go to. Try to choose a restaurant that has a menu offering healthy choices such as grilled fish, meat, and poultry dishes. But keep in mind that restaurant meals tend to have more calories than similar dishes cooked at home, thanks to extra added fat and larger portion sizes. You need to be assertive and order your meal the way you want it. Here are a few tips:

- Ask that the fish, meat, or poultry either be grilled without butter or oil, or prepared lightly with only a little oil or butter.

- Ask for only a half portion of pasta.

- Choose tomato-based pasta dishes rather than creamy ones.

- Stick with broth-based soups such as vegetable, minestrone, lentil, and bean.

- If you have a choice of sides, order steamed veggies or salad instead of mashed potatoes or frites.

- Ask for salsa with a baked potato instead of butter, sour cream, cheese, or bacon.

- Order sandwiches without butter, mayonnaise, or "special sauce."

- Order salad dressings, sauces, and sour cream on the side. That way you can control how much you use.

- Don't eat it all—take half your meal home. Ask the server to bring a doggie bag with your meal. When the meal is served, portion off half right away.

- Instead of ordering one large entree, order two appetizers, or an appetizer and a salad, as your meal. Or consider sharing an entree with a friend.

- Cut down on starchy side dishes. Skip the bread if the meal comes with rice, potato, or pasta. Or ask for extra vegetables instead of the potatoes or rice.

What is okay to eat in a Thai restaurant?

Asian cuisine, with the exception of Japanese, can be tricky because so many dishes are stir-fried in a hefty amount of oil. Many Thai dishes are also made with high-fat coconut milk. You need to order carefully and watch your portion size. Here are a few tips:

- Choose the lighter stir-fried dishes over dishes made with coconut milk, cashews, peanuts, and peanut sauce.

- Order cold fresh salad rolls instead of fried spring rolls.

- Choose lower fat starters, including clear soups such as tom yam goong (hot and sour shrimp soup), green mango salad, and seafood salad.

- Avoid dishes with fried noodles (mee krob, radnar talay) and fried rice. Instead, choose lower fat dishes such as satay, grilled, or sautéed fish, meat, or chicken (but keep portions small) and sautéed tofu.

- Order steamed rice instead of oily pad thai as a side.

- Use your portion size skills to visualize what your serving should look like on the plate.

- Use chopsticks to slow your eating pace.

How do I manage a long driving trip?

You need to plan for your road trip, with or without the kids, by packing your No-Fail Diet snacks. Pack a cooler with single servings of yogurt, fresh fruit, raw vegetable sticks, and plenty of bottled water. Bring snack-sized zip-lock bags filled with dried apricots and almonds. But limit your munching to your designated snack times. Try to plan your route so that you can stop somewhere for meals, before you get too hungry. If your driving trip starts in the morning from home, I recommend packing lunch for everyone.

What should I order in a fast-food restaurant?

Most fast-food restaurants have low-fat items on their menu boards. Best choices include grilled chicken sandwiches, grilled fish burgers, and veggie burgers (skip the processed cheese). If the bun is too large, don't eat it all. Order a side salad instead of french fries. Entree salads are another option, but avoid ones with fatty toppings such as bacon, cheese, or deep-fried tortilla chips. Ask for calorie-reduced dressing to be served on the side so you use only the amount your meal plan calls for. Some fast-food restaurants serve chili, an alternative to a sandwich.

Staying on Track

What should I do if I have a sweet craving?

First, ask yourself why you are hankering for something sweet. Did you miss a meal or wait too long to eat? Did you let your blood sugar drop too low by forgetting to eat your planned snack? Sweet cravings are often a sign of hunger or low blood sugar. The easiest way to prevent them is to eat every 3 to 4 hours.

We all crave sweets from time to time, especially if we know they're close at hand—sometimes just knowing that sweets are readily available makes you think about them. You may need to clean out your kitchen cupboards and get rid of the cookies and candies. And don't forget about the treats in the freezer, too.

To satisfy a sweet craving without putting a dent in your calorie intake, try sipping on a mug of tea with milk and honey. Try flavoured teas such as black currant, orange spice, or mango. You might also try instant light hot chocolate made with hot water. It has only 45 calories per cup and it's a good source of calcium. Hot beverages can help you manage cravings because, compared with eating a couple of cookies, it takes you longer to consume them. By the time your mug is empty, the craving has passed.

What happens if I get off track?

You're human. That means you're bound to go off your plan occasionally. The most important thing you can do is move forward. Do not berate yourself. Do not say to yourself, "The rest of the day is a writeoff." Just get right back on your No-Fail Diet meal plan. One lapse won't make any difference to the scale. But if you let them accumulate, they will show up. You need to remind yourself of all the positive changes you have made so far. One little slip is not going to undo any of those changes. Just move past it.

Weighing Yourself

How fast will I lose weight on the No-Fail Diet?

The No-Fail Diet meal plans are designed to help you safely lose up to 2 pounds (1 kg) each week. Depending on which calorie level you choose in Phase 2, you can lose anywhere from 1/2 to 2 pounds (0.2 to 1 kg) every week. Research shows that losing at this rate is safe, effective, and far more likely to be permanent. If you find you're losing weight more slowly than you'd like, increase your exercise or drop down to the lower calorie level.

How often should I weigh myself?

While you are losing weight on the No-Fail Diet, weigh yourself once per week on the same day, first thing in the morning. Write down your weekly weight on the 12-Week Body Measurement Tracker found in Appendix 1. I don't recommend that you weigh-in every day. It's normal for your weight to fluctuate daily from fluid retention. Seeing these natural increases on the scale can lead to frustration and disappointment.

Why do I always weigh more on Monday mornings than I do on Friday mornings?

This is a common complaint among many of my clients. And the reason is usually the same—overeating on the weekend. Straying from the No-Fail Diet on the weekend—larger meals, drinking alcohol, a few extra snacks—will cause your body to gain fluid. It's water weight that's showing up on the scale on Monday morning. If you make a habit of eating a little more each weekend, your rate of weight loss will slow down. You'll end up playing catch-up during the week to lose those pounds and a couple of extra. Then the following weekend, you'll put a couple more back on. To achieve steady progress on the No-Fail Diet, you need to be consistent with your eating habits on the weekend. You can't view Saturday and Sunday as vacation days from your diet.

Why have I stopped losing weight despite following the plan closely?

If your weight loss has come to a halt, yet you have been faithfully following the No-Fail Diet and haven't changed your exercise or any other lifestyle factors, you have reached a weight-loss plateau. Plateaus are frustrating but they are a natural part of the weight-loss process. They often occur when you reach a weight that you have not been below for quite some time. As you lose weight, your body requires fewer calories and your rate of weight loss may temporarily slow down.

It takes persistence and consistency to break through a plateau, but you can do it. The key is not giving up. If you say to yourself it doesn't matter what I eat because my weight isn't budging, you'll never break though that number on the scale. I do not advise that you eat less food in order to speed up your weight loss. Instead, the best way to work through a plateau is to notch up your exercise to burn more calories. If you've been doing the same workout routine for months, it's time to challenge your body. Consider cross-training by adding different types of cardiovascular workouts to your weekly routine. If you are not doing so already, add one cardio interval training session each week. (For more information on interval training, see page 34 in Chapter 2.) Or it might be time to add strength-training exercises to your program. Strength training helps build more muscles to rev up calorie burning.

Supplements

Do I need to take a multivitamin supplement while losing weight?

I recommend that healthy people take a multivitamin and mineral supplement whether they are losing weight or not. While you should always strive to eat right first, a multivitamin helps ensure that you are meeting your daily requirements for folic acid (a B vitamin), B12, vitamin D, and iron—nutrients that can be challenging for many people to get from food alone. The No-Fail Diet requires you to reduce your calorie intake. Eating less food means you will also be consuming fewer vitamins and minerals. With the possible exceptions of calcium, vitamin D, and iron, the No-Fail Diet is designed to give you the nutrients you need. Despite this, I still recommend a daily multivitamin supplement. (For information on choosing a supplement, see page 82 in Chapter 4.)

Do I need to take a calcium supplement?

Depending on your age and what calorie level you are following, the answer may be yes.

On page 84 in Chapter 4 I have outlined how much calcium you need each day, who should take a supplement, and how much of the mineral you need to supplement your diet with.

Are there any supplements I can take to speed up my metabolism?

No. There are many supplements marketed to help burn fat and speed metabolism, but the truth is that they don't work. And some can be harmful. The few products that did have positive results in small studies were conducted among people who also exercised and followed a calorie-reduced diet. There is no magic bullet when it comes to losing weight. The only surefire way to rev up your metabolism is to start strength training.

Health Concerns

Should I follow the No-Fail Diet if I have high blood cholesterol?

Absolutely. In fact, this is the very same type of diet I recommend for my clients who have elevated cholesterol levels. Losing weight alone will help bring down your cholesterol reading. But the No-Fail Diet teaches you how to choose foods that are low in saturated fat and trans fats, two types of fat that tend to raise cholesterol levels. When making choices from the Starchy Foods group, select foods high in soluble fibre— oatmeal, oat bran cereal, and Kellogg's All-Bran Buds, for example. Include nuts, especially almonds, as part of your daily Fats and Oils servings. Both soluble fibre and almonds help lower cholesterol levels.

Is the No-Fail Diet safe for me if I have high blood pressure?

Yes. Losing weight is an important strategy to lower your blood pressure. But the types of foods you eat each day can also help reduce your blood pressure numbers. Foods that contain calcium, magnesium, and potassium are part of a low-fat diet that lowers blood pressure. And all these foods are prescribed in the No-Fail Diet. To get these nutrients, make sure your daily diet includes 2 or 3 low-fat dairy servings, 2 servings of fruit, and at least 4 servings of vegetables. Include legumes and nuts in your diet four times per week (legumes are in the Protein Foods group). You'll also find information on managing your sodium intake on page 65 in Chapter 3.

If you are taking medication for high blood pressure, monitor your blood pressure regularly as you lose weight. If you find it is getting too low, or you feel light headed, speak with your doctor.

Should I follow the No-Fail Diet if I have type 2 diabetes?

If you have type 2 diabetes and you are not taking medication, this diet is absolutely safe to follow. Losing weight can help you reduce your blood sugar. The foods recommended on the No-Fail Diet are low in refined sugars and many are high in fibre and should be included in any diet to manage diabetes. The No-Fail Diet meal plans show you how to space out your food servings over the course of the day, another important strategy for managing blood sugar.

If you have type 2 diabetes and you are taking a medication that lowers your blood sugar, speak with your doctor or dietitian first. You should *not* follow Phase 1, which eliminates starchy foods at lunch and dinner, but Phase 2 is appropriate for you. Just be sure to eat your meals and snacks at regular intervals to prevent a low blood sugar reaction. Make sure you monitor your blood sugar level regularly.

Beverages

How much water should I drink while losing weight?

If you're female, you need to drink 9 cups (2.2 litres) of water each day to stay adequately hydrated. If you are male, you need 13 cups (3 litres). With the exception of alcoholic beverages, all beverages count toward your daily water requirements: water, fruit juice, vegetable juice, milk, soy milk, coffee, tea, herbal tea, and soft drinks. However, the No-Fail Diet is intended to help you lose weight, so don't waste calories on sugary fruit juice and soft drinks.

May I drink fruit juice?

You may drink fruit juice once per day, provided it is unsweetened and you have only 1/2 cup (125 ml), 1 Fruit serving. The rest of your fruit should come from fresh or dried fruit to boost your fibre intake. If you do drink fruit juice, have it with breakfast, since the vitamin C it contains helps your body absorb more iron from grains.

Where do coffee and tea fit in?

Coffee and tea count toward your daily water requirements. Both beverages may be consumed during the day, with and between meals. Avoid using cream in your coffee and tea, and limit the sugar you add to 1 teaspoon (5 ml). If you drink café lattes, made with milk, you need to treat that as a Milk and Milk Alternative serving also. You'll find guidelines for caffeine consumption on page 71 in Chapter 3.

May I drink diet pop?

Yes, but I advise you to limit your intake to no more than 1 serving a day. Diet soft drinks contain many chemical additives, including phosphoric acid, a substance that may upset calcium balance in the body if consumed in high quantities.

Condiments

May I add salt to foods?

Yes, but do so sparingly. The most important strategy for keeping your daily sodium intake under the daily upper limit of 2300 milligrams is limiting your intake of processed foods. The majority of sodium we consume each day comes from processed foods and restaurant foods. Only about 11% of the sodium we consume comes from the salt shaker. However, if you're used to shaking salt on your foods, it's a good idea to break the habit. Try using lemon juice, herbs, spices, and salt substitutes such as Mrs. Dash to flavour your foods.

May I use condiments such as ketchup, barbecue sauce, and mustard?

Condiments such as mustard, hot sauce, vinegar, and salsa may be used to flavour foods without measuring because they are either calorie-free or very low in calories. You may also use barbecue sauce and ketchup, but limit how much you use to 1 or 2 tablespoons (15 to 25 ml) since they contain sugar. If you use stir-fry sauces to spice up your meals, choose calorie-reduced versions and use no more than 2 tablespoons (25 ml). Calorie-reduced peanut sauces generally provide 50 calories per 2 tablespoons (25 ml) and should be treated as 1 Fats and Oils serving.

Foods and Food Groups

Do I need to weigh and measure my foods?

Yes. Monitoring your portion size is a key to losing weight and keeping it off. I strongly recommend that for the first two weeks on the No-Fail Diet you weigh and measure your foods so that you know how much you're eating. Measuring your foods will give you a good sense of what a certain amount of food looks like on your plate. After a few weeks, you won't need to measure your foods. Instead, you can eyeball your portion sizes. On pages 14 to 16 in Chapter 1, you'll learn two techniques to help you judge the amount of food you're eating.

How often may I treat myself to a high-calorie food that's off the plan?

During Phase 1, the 2-Week Quick Start Meal Plan, splurges are not allowed: You are required to be strict with your diet for two weeks. In Phase 2, you may include a treat once per week. Your treat may be any high-calorie food you like—a few chocolate chip cookies, a small bowl of ice cream, an order of french fries, even a meal of macaroni and cheese. You are to enjoy an indulgence once each week so that you don't feel deprived.

Why is cheese counted as a Protein Food serving, rather than as a Milk and Milk Alternatives serving?

I have included part-skim cheese in the Protein food group because it is a very good source of protein. One serving (1 ounce or 30 grams) of low-fat cheese provides roughly 7 grams of protein. That's the same amount of protein you'll find in 1 serving of all the other foods listed in the Protein food group. It is true that hard cheese is an excellent source of calcium, but you'd have to eat more than 1 ounce (30 grams) to get the same amount of calcium found in 1 serving of milk—and that means more calories. (Cottage cheese is much lower in calcium than hard cheese.) Counting part-skim cheese as a Protein food also helps you increase your calcium intake beyond what you consume from the recommended servings of Milk and Milk Alternatives.

May I eat frozen dinners on the No-Fail Diet?

If you are pressed for time, you may use low-fat frozen dinners occasionally. But I don't want you to rely on them. Although many frozen meals are low in fat, all have far more sodium than does a home-cooked meal of fresh foods. When buying a frozen dinner, choose one with no more than 3 grams of fat per 100 calories and no more than 600 milligrams of sodium. Most 300-calorie frozen dinners count as 2 to 3 Protein Food servings, 2 Starchy Food servings, and 1 Fats and Oils serving. You will need to supplement your frozen meal with vegetables.

Nutrition Labels

How will nutrition labels help me determine what 1 Starchy Food serving is?

Reading the Nutrition Facts box on food packaging can be a useful way to determine appropriate serving sizes—you might want to know how many crackers count as 1 No-Fail Diet Starchy Food serving, or how much ready-to-eat breakfast cereal you should have for your morning meal. One No-Fail Diet Starchy Food serving has 15 grams of carbohydrate and roughly 65 to 85 calories. So if the label on the box of whole-grain snack crackers tells you that eight crackers have 30 grams of carbohydrate and 160 calories, then eight crackers count as 2 Starchy Food servings.

How will nutrition labels help me determine what 1 Fats and Oils serving is?

One No-Fail Diet Fats and Oils serving has 4 grams of fat and 45 calories. Use this information when reading nutrition labels on frozen dinners or prepared foods that have oils added. For example, if the label on a frozen dinner of chicken breast, rice, and vegetables states 6 grams of fat, there are 1 1/2 Fats and Oils servings already in this meal.

Keep in mind that Protein Foods such as lean meat, fish, eggs, and part-skim cheese contain some fat naturally. The grams of fat on labels of packaged foods with these ingredients will include this naturally occurring fat.

How will nutrition labels help me determine if a food has too much sodium?

When it comes to choosing foods based on sodium content, you need to read the percentage of daily value (% DV) for sodium. The % DV is stated for 1 serving of the food and is based on an intake of 2400 milligrams. Foods with a % DV of 25% or more are high in sodium. You shouldn't eat more than 2 servings of high-sodium foods per day. Foods with a % DV of 5% or less for sodium are low in sodium.

Exercise

Will strength training make me look too muscular?

No. Many women are afraid that weight training will make them look bulky. Women don't have enough of the male hormone testosterone to create large, bulky muscles.

For the average woman, strength training results in relatively small increases in muscle size—certainly not enough to show up on the scale. But strength training has enormous benefits for women (and men), including a well-toned body, enhanced strength and power, and improved physical performance. And there are health benefits—stronger bones, reduced risk of osteoporosis, and less susceptibility to injury, to name just a few.

I don't have 30 minutes a day to devote to a cardio workout. Any suggestions?

You don't have to do your 30-minute cardio workout all at one time. If time is a factor, you may break up your cardio into two 15-minute sessions or even three bouts of 10 minutes. At the end of the day you will still burn the same number of calories. If you are going to do shorter duration cardio workouts, consider increasing their intensity to help you burn even more calories over the course of the day. If you need to break up your strength program into manageable amounts of time, you can do that, too. You might do your upper body exercises in the morning and your lower body and core exercises in the evenings.

Are there certain exercises I can do to lose fat from my hips and thighs?

Unfortunately, you can't melt away fat from those trouble spots with specific exercises. You can only lose body fat by reducing your calorie intake and increasing your calorie expenditure by exercising. Where you lose your body fat depends on your genes. In general, losing weight around the abdomen is easier than losing from the hips and thighs. However, certain lower-body strength exercises can tone the muscles of your upper legs, making them appear longer and leaner. If you work out at a gym, ask a certified personal trainer to show you how to do lower-body strength exercises.

Endnotes

1 Getting Ready to Start the No-Fail Diet

1. de Castro, JM. The time of day of food intake influences overall intake in humans. *J Nutr* 2004, 134(1):104–11.

2. Romon, M, JL Edme, C Boulenguez, JL Lescroart, and P Frimat. Circadian variation of diet-induced thermogenesis. *Am J Clin Nutr* 1993, 57(4):476–80.

3. Feskanich, D, WC Willett, MJ Stampfer, and GA Colditz. Protein consumption and bone fractures in women. *Am J Epidemiol* 1996, 143(5):472–79.

4. Wadden, TA, RI Berkowitz, LG Womble, DB Sarwer, S Phelan, RK Cato, LA Hesson, SY Osei, R Kaplan, and AJ Stunkard. Randomized trial of lifestyle modification and pharmacotherapy for obesity. *N Eng J Med* 2005, 353(20):2111–20.

5. Klem, ML, RR Wing, MT McGuire, HM Seagle, and JO Hill. A descriptive study of individuals successful at long-term maintenance of substantial weight loss. *Am J Clin Nutr* 1997, 66(2):239–46.

6. Wamsteker, EW, R Geenen, J Iestra, JK Larsen, PM Zelissen, and WA van Staveren. Obesity-related beliefs predict weight loss after an 8-week low-calorie diet. *J Am Diet Assoc* 2005, 105(3):441–44.

2 Getting and Staying Active

1. Klem, ML, RR Wing, MT McGuire, HM Seagle, and JO Hill. A descriptive study of individuals successful at long-term maintenance of substantial weight loss. *Am J Clin Nutr* 1997, 66(2):239–46.

2. Winett, RA, and RN Carpinelli. Potential health-related benefits of resistance training. *Prev Med* 2001, 33(5):503–13.

3 Foods for Health and Longevity

1. Albert, CM, K Oh, W Whang, JE Manson, CU Chae, MJ Stampfer, WC Willett, and FB Hu. Dietary alpha-linolenic acid intake and risk of sudden cardiac death and coronary heart disease. *Circulation* 2005, 112(21):3232–38.

2. Erkkila, AT, DM Herrington, D Mozaffarian, and AH Lichtenstein. Cereal fiber and whole-grain intake are associated with reduced progression of coronary-artery atherosclerosis in postmenopausal women with coronary artery disease. *Am Heart J* 2005, 150(1):94–101.

3. Boschmann, M, J Steiniger, U Hille, J Tank, F Adams, AM Sharma, S Klaus, FC Luft, and J Jordan. Water-induced thermogenesis. *J Clin Endocrinol Metab* 2003, 88(12):6015–19.

4. Mahmud, A, and J Feely. Acute effect of caffeine on arterial stiffness and aortic pressure waveform. *Hypertension* 2001, 38(2):227–31.

Subject Index

Recipe Index